D0771336

Controversies in the Treatment of Prostate Cancer

Frontiers of Radiation Therapy and Oncology

Vol. 41

Series Editors

J.L. Meyer San Francisco, Calif.
W. Hinkelbein Berlin

10th International Symposium on Special Aspects of Radiotherapy,
Berlin, September 2–8, 2006

Controversies in the Treatment of Prostate Cancer

Volume Editors

L. Moser Berlin

M. Schostak Berlin

K. Miller Berlin

W. Hinkelbein Berlin

20 figures, 2 in color, and 15 tables, 2008

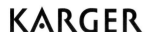

Basel · Freiburg · Paris · London · New York ·
Bangalore · Bangkok · Shanghai · Singapore · Tokyo · Sydney

Frontiers of Radiation Therapy and Oncology

Founded 1968 by J.M. Vaeth, San Francisco, Calif.

Dr. Lutz Moser
Prof. Wolfgang Hinkelbein

Department of Radiooncology and Radiotherapy
Charité – Campus Benjamin Franklin
Berlin (Germany)

PD Dr. Martin Schostak
Prof. Kurt Miller

Department of Urology
Charité – Campus Benjamin Franklin
Berlin (Germany)

Library of Congress Cataloging-in-Publication Data

International Symposium on Special Aspects of Radiotherapy (10th : 2006 : Berlin, Germany)
  Controversies in the treatment of prostate cancer / volume editors, L.
Moser ... [et al.]. ; 10th International Symposium on Special Aspects of
Radiotherapy, Berlin, September 2-8, 2006.
    p. ; cm. -- (Frontiers of radiation therapy and oncology, ISSN 0071-9676 ; v. 41)
  Includes bibliographical references and indexes.
  ISBN 978-3-8055-8524-8 (hard cover : alk. paper)
  1. Prostate--Cancer--Radiotherapy--Congresses. I. Moser, L. (Lutz) II. Title. III. Series.
  [DNLM: 1. Prostatic Neoplasms--radiotherapy--Congresses. 2.
Hormones--therapeutic use--Congresses. 3. Neoplasm Recurrence,
Local--therapy--Congresses. 4. Prostatectomy--Congresses. 5. Prostatic
Neoplasms--surgery--Congresses. W3 FR935 v. 41 2008 / WJ 762 I61c 2008]
  RC280.P7I565 2006
  362.196'99463--dc22

                                                              2008003793

Bibliographic Indices. This publication is listed in bibliographic services, including Current Contents® and PubMed/
MEDLINE.

© Copyright 2008 by S. Karger AG, P.O. Box, CH–4009 Basel (Switzerland)
www.karger.com
Printed in Switzerland on acid-free and non-aging paper (ISO 9706) by Reinhardt Druck, Basel
ISSN 0071–9676
ISBN 978–3–8055–8524–8

Contents

Localized and Locally Advanced Prostate Cancer

1   **Prostate Cancer and Active Surveillance**
          Abrahamsson, PA (Malmö)

7   **Radical Prostatectomy in the 21st Century – The Gold Standard for Localized and Locally Advanced Prostate Cancer**
          Schostak, M; Miller, K; Schrader, M (Berlin)

15   **Radiotherapy as Primary Treatment Modality**
          Sia, M; Rosewall, T; Warde, P (Toronto, Ont.)

26   **Combined Radiotherapy and Hormonal Therapy in the Treatment of Prostate Cancer**
          Boehmer, D (Berlin)

32   **Postoperative Adjuvant Radiotherapy – Standard of Care?**
          Bottke, D; Wiegel, T (Ulm)

39   **Adjuvant Hormonal Treatment – The Bicalutamide Early Prostate Cancer Program**
          Wirth, MP; Hakenberg, OW; Froehner, M (Dresden)

49   **Hormone Therapy for Prostate Cancer – Immediate Initiation**
          Schostak, M; Miller, K; Schrader, M (Berlin)

Lymph Node-Positive Prostate Cancer

58   **Lymphadenectomy in Prostate Cancer. Radio-Guided Lymph Node Mapping: An Adequate Staging Method**
          Winter, A; Wawroschek, F (Oldenburg)

68   **Radiotherapy in Lymph Node-Positive Prostate Cancer Patients – A Potential Cure? Single Institutional Experience Regarding Outcome and Side Effects**
          Goldner, G; Pötter, R (Vienna)

Biochemical Recurrence after Therapy

77   **Radiotherapy in Biochemical Recurrences after Surgery for Prostate Cancer**
Höcht, S; Lohm, G; Moser, L; Hinkelbein, W (Berlin)

86   **Recurrence following Radiotherapy**
Desgrandchamps, F (Paris)

Hormone-Refractory and Metastatic Prostate Cancer

93   **Secondary Hormonal Manipulation**
Merseburger, AS; Belka, C; Behmenburg, K; Stenzl, A (Tübingen)

103   **Chemotherapy in Hormone-Refractory Prostate Cancer**
Wolff, JM (Bad Mergentheim)

108   **A Randomized Phase II Trial Comparing Weekly Taxotere plus Prednisone versus Prednisone Alone in Androgen-Independent Prostate Cancer**
Fosså, SD (Oslo)

117   **Hormone-Refractory and Metastatic Prostate Cancer – Palliative Radiotherapy**
Moser, L; Schubert, T; Hinkelbein, W (Berlin)

126   **Author Index**
127   **Subject Index**

Moser L, Schostak M, Miller K, Hinkelbein W (eds): Controversies in the Treatment of
Prostate Cancer. Front Radiat Ther Oncol. Basel, Karger, 2008, vol 41, pp 1–6

Prostate Cancer and Active Surveillance

Per-Anders Abrahamsson

Department of Urology, Malmö University Hospital, Malmö, Sweden

Abstract

This review outlines the different treatment options in localized prostate cancer. This information can be considered alongside other important factors, such as the individual patient's values and situation as well as the potential impact of treatment on his quality of life, in the treatment decision-making process. Taking all these factors into consideration, the data support active surveillance as an appropriate choice in patients with well or moderately differentiated, low-volume prostate cancer who have a life expectancy of less than 10 years. Men with higher-grade tumors and longer life expectancy may be at excess risk of death from prostate cancer managed with active surveillance.

Prostate cancer is a major cause of death among men in European countries, with nearly 202,100 cases and 68,200 deaths in the EU in 2004 [1]. The incidence varies considerably between countries and appears to be increasing because of more frequent and better diagnostic tests, an ageing population and probably a true increase in the occurrence of the disease [2]. There are no obvious strategies for prevention, so screening and early detection have been considered as possible interventions to reduce the number of deaths [3].

The increase in the incidence of prostate cancer raises the possibility that many cases detected by prostate-specific antigen (PSA) testing are overtreated. In other words, many patients may not become symptomatic despite being left untreated. The challenge of managing early prostate cancer is to differentiate patients with clinically relevant cancers from those whose 'disease' is destined to be merely an incidental histological phenomenon.

The Natural History of Prostate Cancer and Diagnostic Tests

The natural history of prostate cancer is not fully established. It is well known, however, that the disease is often indolent. It is slow growing in many cases, and there is a long phase during which it remains undiscovered. This long latent phase is potentially advantageous for screening, but it appears that some tumors are very slow growing and may never become clinically important [4, 5]. Men with such tumors often die from another cause [6]. Although the outcome varies strongly with age at diagnosis and with Gleason score, it is interesting that the predicted 15-year prostate cancer mortality rate in men with Gleason score 2–4 cancer is approximately 4–7%, compared with 27–73% mortality from other causes [6]. The mortality rate in men with very localized tumors is little different from that in other men [6, 7]. The relatively benign course of many tumors means that, in most cases, the benefits of treatment might not outweigh its side effects.

There are, in principle, 2 tests that may be used in mass screening: PSA and digital rectal examination (DRE). The PSA test is simple, cheap, safe and acceptable. However, prostate biopsy, which is required to investigate positive results, is less acceptable and carries significant risks. The accuracy (sensitivity and specificity) of the PSA test is difficult to determine [8]. There is no gold standard against which to test it, because prostate biopsy itself may miss 10–30% of cases. Also, biopsies are not normally performed on men with a negative PSA test, so it is difficult to assess the number of false-negative tests and thus to measure the sensitivity of the PSA test. Testing does not differentiate between relatively harmless tumors and those that are likely to be fatal; therefore, the PSA test is not specific for clinically important disease. DRE is less acceptable and less accurate (that is, it has lower sensitivity and specificity) than PSA testing [8].

Comprehensive guidelines for the management of prostate cancer were recently published by the European Association of Urology (available online at www.uroweb.org).

Treatment Options for Localized Prostate Cancer

Current management options for localized prostate cancer include radical prostatectomy, external beam radiotherapy or brachytherapy (the insertion of radioactive seeds into the prostate gland), active surveillance and hormone therapy. However, the benefits of these options have yet to be adequately documented in randomized controlled trials.

There is evidence from 1 trial, the fourth Scandinavian Prostatic Cancer Group study (SPCG-4) [9], that compared with watchful waiting, radical surgery may reduce prostate cancer deaths: at 10 years, there were fewer deaths among men who had undergone radical prostatectomy than among those who had undergone watchful waiting (relative risk 0.56, p = 0.01) [10]. At a median follow-up of 8.2 years, there was a small but significant (p = 0.04) reduction in the 10-year overall mortality rate in the radical prostatectomy group (relative risk 0.74) [10]. In addition, a significant reduction in the risk of distant metastases emerged at 10 years (relative risk 0.60, p = 0.004). There is no evidence from randomized controlled trials that radiotherapy is better than watchful waiting [8]. The same is currently valid for external beam radiotherapy and brachytherapy.

Several years will elapse before mature results are available from randomized controlled trials of treatment of localized prostate cancer, including the SPCG-4, the Prostate Cancer Intervention versus Observation Trial [11] and the Prostate Testing for Cancer and Treatment study [12].

Evidence of the benefit of active surveillance in low- and intermediate-risk patients is discussed below.

Active Surveillance
Active surveillance comprises active monitoring, with tailored treatment only if there is evidence of disease progression. Suitable patients have only 1 or 2 biopsy cores with cancer, Gleason score 6 or less, PSA 15 ng/ml or less, PSA density less than 0.2 ng/ml/cm^3 and clinical stage T1c or T2 [13].

Data from retrospective cohort studies and case series support active surveillance as an appropriate choice in patients with well or moderately differentiated, low-volume prostate cancer who have a life expectancy of less than 10 years. However, men with higher-grade tumors and longer life expectancy may be at excess risk of death from prostate cancer managed with active surveillance [5–7, 14–16]. This information can be considered alongside other important factors, such as the individual patient's values and situation as well as the potential impact of treatment on his quality of life, in the treatment decision-making process.

The prognosis for men with localized prostate cancer can be excellent and active surveillance can achieve survival rates similar to those of more aggressive treatment [5–7, 9, 14, 17]. Screen-detected cancers are mostly of this type.

A prospective phase II study of active surveillance with selective delayed intervention was initiated in 1995 [18, 19]. Management was initially surveillance; patients who had a PSA doubling time of 2 years or less or had a grade progression on rebiopsy were offered radical intervention. The remaining patients were closely monitored. The cohort comprised 299 patients aged 70 years or more who had low-risk prostate cancer (PSA <10 ng/ml, Gleason score <6 or stage <T2a) or intermediate-risk prostate cancer (PSA 10–20 ng/ml, Gleason score 7 or stage T2b/c). The median PSA doubling time was 7 years, and 42% of the cohort had a PSA doubling time of more than 10 years. Most patients remain on surveillance.

Table 1. Risk of complications following surgery or radiotherapy

Risk	Surgery, %	Radiotherapy, %
Death	0.48[1]; 0.37–0.56[2]	<1
Erectile dysfunction 2 years after surgery	79.6[3]	61.5
Incontinence	9.6	3.5

Adapted with permission from Slaughter et al. [22].
[1] Data from Alibhai et al. [20]
[2] Data from Lu-Yao et al. [21]
[3] The risk may be as low as 32% with bilateral nerve-sparing surgery by experts [23]. It is not known whether this rate can be generally achieved.

At 8 years, the overall actuarial survival is 85%, and the disease-specific survival is 99%. To date, this study has shown that almost all men with low-risk prostate cancer managed in this manner will die of unrelated causes. The approach of active surveillance with selective delayed intervention based on PSA doubling time and repeat biopsy represents a practical compromise between radical therapy for all patients (which results in overtreatment of indolent disease) and watchful waiting with palliative therapy only (which results in undertreatment of aggressive disease).

Radical Treatment of Localized Prostate Cancer
Radical treatment (surgery or radiotherapy) can be harmful as well as beneficial. The principal adverse events following surgery are sexual dysfunction and incontinence. Surgery is fatal in approximately 0.5% of cases [20, 21] and radiotherapy can cause sexual dysfunction, urinary symptoms and diarrhea or rectal bleeding (table 1). Furthermore, there are important potential harms at the population level. These harms can arise from the diversion of health care resources from other, more effective treatments towards an ineffective or poorly performed screening or early detection program.

Conclusion

This review has outlined the different treatment options in localized prostate cancer. This information can be considered alongside other important factors, such as the individual patient's values and situation as well as the potential impact of treatment on his quality of life, in the treatment decision-making process. Taking all these factors into consideration, the data support active surveillance as an appropriate choice in patients with well or moderately differentiated, low-volume prostate cancer who have a life expectancy of less than 10 years. Men with higher-grade tumors and longer life expectancy may be at excess risk of death from prostate cancer managed with active surveillance.

In the future, translational research aimed at identifying the molecular profiles of prostate tumors will lead to a better understanding of the key pathways and molecular events leading to prostate cancer and to the identification of better prognostic markers to select patients who are suitable for active surveillance versus those with aggressive tumors who are candidates for radical treatment.

References

1 Boyle P, Ferlay J: Cancer incidence and mortality in Europe, 2004. Ann Oncol 2005;16:481–488.
2 Schersten T, Baile MA, Asua J, Jonsson E: Prostate Cancer Screening: Evidence Synthesis and Update (INAHTA Joint Project). Vitoria-Gasteiz, Basque Office for Health Technology Assessment, Health Department Basque Government (OSTEBA), 1999.
3 Council of Europe: Recommendation No. R(94)11 on Screening as a Tool of Preventive Medicine. Strasbourg, Council of Europe, 1994.
4 Johansson JE: Expectant management of early stage prostatic cancer: Swedish experience. J Urol 1994;152:1753–1756.
5 Chodak GW, Thisted RA, Gerber GS, et al: Results of conservative management of clinically localized prostate cancer. N Engl J Med 1994;330:242–248.
6 Albertsen PC, Hanley JA, Gleason DF, Barry MJ: Competing risk analysis of men aged 55 to 74 years at diagnosis managed conservatively for clinically localized prostate cancer. JAMA 1998;280:975–980.
7 Albertsen PC, Fryback DG, Storer BE, Kolon TF, Fine J: Long-term survival among men with conservatively treated localized prostate cancer. JAMA 1995;274:626–631.
8 Harris R, Lohr KN: Screening for prostate cancer: an update of the evidence for the U.S. Preventive Services Task Force. Ann Intern Med 2002;137:917–929.
9 Holmberg L, Bill-Axelson A, Helgesen F, et al: A randomized trial comparing radical prostatectomy with watchful waiting in early prostate cancer. N Engl J Med 2002;347:781–789.
10 Bill-Axelson A, Holmberg L, Ruutu M, Häggman M, Andersson SO, Bratell S, Spångberg A, Busch C, Nordling S, Garmo H, Palmgren J, Adami HO, Norlén BJ, Johansson JE, Scandinavian Prostate Cancer Group Study No. 4: Radical prostatectomy versus watchful waiting in early prostate cancer. N Engl J Med 2005;352:1977–1984.
11 Wilt TJ, Brawer MK: Early intervention or expectant management for prostate cancer. The Prostate Cancer Intervention Versus Observation Trial (PIVOT): a randomized trial comparing radical prostatectomy with expectant management for the treatment of clinically localized prostate cancer. Semin Urol 1995;13:130–136.
12 Donovan J, Hamdy F, Neal D, et al: Prostate Testing for Cancer and Treatment (ProtecT) feasibility study. Health Technol Assess 2003;7:1–88.
13 Roemeling S, Roobol MJ, Postma R, et al: Management and survival of screen-detected prostate cancer patients who might have been suitable for active surveillance. Eur Urol 2006;50:475–482.
14 Johansson JE, Holmberg L, Johansson S, Bergstrom R, Adami HO: Fifteen-year survival in prostate cancer: a prospective, population-based study in Sweden. JAMA 1997;277:467–471.
15 Brasso K, Friis S, Juel K, Jørgensen T, Iversen P: Mortality of patients with clinically localized prostate cancer treated with observation for 10 years or longer: a population based registry study. J Urol 1999;161:524–528.
16 Aus G, Hugosson J, Norlén L: Long-term survival and mortality in prostate cancer treated with noncurative intent. J Urol 1995;154:460–465.
17 Sandblom G, Dufmats M, Varenhorst E: Long-term survival in a Swedish population-based cohort of men with prostate cancer. Urology 2000;56:442–447.

18 Klotz L: Active surveillance with selective delayed intervention using PSA doubling time for good risk prostate cancer. Eur Urol 2005;47:16–21.

19 Klotz L, Nam R: Active surveillance with selective delayed intervention for favourable risk prostate cancer: clinical experience and a 'number needed to treat' analysis. Eur Urol Suppl 2006;5:479–486.

20 Alibhai SMH, Leach M, Tomlinson G, et al: 30-day mortality and major complications after radical prostatectomy: influence of age and comorbidity. J Natl Cancer Inst 2005;97:1525–1532.

21 Lu-Yao GL, Albertsen P, Warren J, Yao S-L: Effect of age and surgical approach on complications and short-term mortality after radical prostatectomy – a population-based study. Urology 1999;54:301–307.

22 Slaughter P, Pinfold S, Laupacis A: Prostate-Specific Antigen (PSA) Screening in Asymptomatic Men. Toronto, Institute for Clinical Evaluative Sciences, 2002.

23 Catalona WJ, Carvalhal GF, Mager DE, Smith DS: Potency, continence and complication rates in 1,870 consecutive radical retropubic prostatectomies. J Urol 1999;162:433–438.

Prof. Per-Anders Abrahamsson
Department of Urology, Malmö University Hospital
SE–205 02 Malmö (Sweden)
Tel. +46 40 33 3749, Fax +46 40 33 7049, E-Mail Per-Anders.Abrahamsson@skane.se

Moser L, Schostak M, Miller K, Hinkelbein W (eds): Controversies in the Treatment of
Prostate Cancer. Front Radiat Ther Oncol. Basel, Karger, 2008, vol 41, pp 7–14

Radical Prostatectomy in the 21st Century – The Gold Standard for Localized and Locally Advanced Prostate Cancer

M. Schostak   K. Miller   M. Schrader

Department of Urology, Charité Universitätsmedizin Berlin, Berlin, Germany

Abstract

Radical prostatectomy for treatment of prostate cancer is a technically sophisticated operation. Simpler therapies have therefore been developed in the course of decades. The decisive advantage of a radical operation is the chance of a cure with minimal collateral damage. It is the only approach that enables precise tumor staging. The 10-year progression-free survival probability is approximately 85% for a localized tumor with negative resection margins. This high cure rate is unsurpassed by competitive treatment modalities. Nowadays, experienced surgeons achieve excellent functional results (for example, recovery of continence and erectile function) with minimum morbidity. Even in the locally advanced stage, results are very good compared to those obtained with other treatment modalities. Pathological staging enables stratified adjuvant therapy based on concrete information. The overall prognosis can thus be significantly improved.   Copyright © 2008 S. Karger AG, Basel

Prostate cancer is the most common male tumor disease in many industrial countries. In Germany, 48,700 new cases were diagnosed in 2002. With more than 11,400 cases per year, prostate cancer is the third most common cause of death in Germany [1]. The broad spectrum of the tumor's aggressiveness and the relatively high median age at diagnosis result in high variability of the natural disease course.

Radical prostatectomy was the first curative therapy for prostate cancer and has been performed for more than 100 years [2–4]. It is a technically very sophisticated operation. In the course of decades, this has led to the development of simpler therapies, whose ideal areas of application are controversially discussed. The following article advocates radical prostatectomy as the gold standard for localized and locally advanced disease stages, especially in younger patients.

Radical Prostatectomy for Localized Prostate Cancer

The decisive advantage of radical prostatectomy is the chance of a cure with minimal collateral damage. It is the only approach that enables precise tumor staging. Extraction of the surgical specimen provides the pathologist with more detailed microscopic information on the aggressiveness and precise dissemination than random sampling.

The principle of radical prostatectomy is complete removal of the cancer-bearing organ. Important endpoints of local cancer control are confirmed organ confinement with negative resection margins and freedom from recurrence. Biochemical recurrence precedes clinical progression by an average of 8 years and cancer-specific mortality by an average of 13 years [5]. The freedom-from-progression rate varies widely in relation to clinical and pathological parameters. Independent clinical prognostic factors are the tumor stage, the Gleason score, the preoperative prostate-specific antigen (PSA) and the patient's age at the time of diagnosis and/or therapy [6–9]. Unfavorable prognostic factors are non-organ-confined disease, perineural or lymphovascular invasion, extracapsular tumor growth, positive resection margins, infiltration of seminal vesicles, lymph node metastases and a high PSA-velocity before the operation [10–15, 40]. The introduction of PSA testing markedly improved patient selection and thus also the overall effectiveness of radical prostatectomy.

The 10-year progression-free survival probability is approximately 85% for a localized tumor with negative resection margins [16]. This high cure rate is unsurpassed by competitive treatment modalities. In the case of localized prostate cancer with negative resection margins, the PSA drops to zero after radical prostatectomy, which enables a particularly subtle follow-up with very early detection of a tumor recurrence. A value below 0.2 ng/ml in at least 2 consecutive controls is assessed as nondetectable [17].

Continence
The probability of regaining continence after surgery is very high nowadays. It depends on 2 factors: (1) the surgeon's experience: recovery of full continence is achieved in 90% of the men treated by very experienced surgeons; (2) the patient's age: the probability of recovering full continence is 95% for patients under 50 years of age, but only 80–85% for those over 70 [18].

Erectile Function

Potency is commonly defined as the ability to achieve erections firm enough for penetration and satisfactory sexual intercourse without using devices or drugs. With suitable selection, the vast majority of operations can preserve potency in patients with a localized tumor. Risk classifications for this selection differ among the centers [10, 11, 14, 19, 20]. Some institutions use rapid intraoperative analysis of resection margins in order to decide whether or not the respective neurovascular bundle must be removed [21, 22]. Potency can be retained in about 85% of younger men (under 60 years of age) with bilateral nerve-sparing surgery, which means that the initial potency level is reached after about 1 year. This probability decreases with age, dropping to 75% in 60- to 70-year-old patients and to 50% in men over 70. The recovery of erectile function is a lengthy process. Partial erections usually only occur 3–6 months after surgery. Improvements may be expected up to 3 years thereafter [23, 24]. Postoperative erection aids like PDE5 inhibitors, intracavernous injection or vacuum pumps improve performance during erectile rehabilitation and should therefore be recommended in clinics that mainly use the nerve-sparing technique [25, 26].

Complications

The complication rate of radical prostatectomy has decreased dramatically during the decades following its introduction. Open retropubic radical prostatectomy still had a transfusion probability of 20–50% a few years ago [27–30]. Improved anesthesia management has now almost completely resolved this problem [31]. The bleeding probability is already markedly lower in laparoscopic prostatectomy due to the intraabdominal gas pressure [32].

In summary, radical prostatectomy in the localized tumor stage offers younger patients decisive advantages: it is the oldest therapy and thus has the longest follow-up period. This advantage is particularly important in view of the slow tumor growth of prostate cancer. Nowadays, experienced surgeons achieve excellent functional results, including the recovery of continence and erectile function.

Radical Prostatectomy in the Locally Advanced Tumor Stage

Non-organ-confined growth, involvement of the seminal vesicles or adjacent organs and lymph node metastases are designated as locally advanced prostate cancer. There are different methods for preoperative classification of the individual risk. The so-called Partin Tables are most commonly used. In the most recent version (2001), the probability of organ-confined growth, seminal vesicle infiltration and lymph node metastases is based on the digital rectal examination, the Gleason score and the preoperative PSA [20].

Surgery in Clinical Stage T3

Clinical detection (that is, rectal palpation) of a non-organ-confined tumor does not necessarily mean that the cancer cannot be excised with negative resection margins during radical prostatectomy. The prognosis for stage pT3 after radical prostatectomy is far better with negative than with positive resection margins [11]. In large series, cancer-specific survival for a clinically detected non-organ-confined tumor is 85–92% after 5 years and 79–82% after 10 years [33, 34]. This observation is independent of any adjuvant (radio)therapy, which significantly improves the results in cases with local non-organ confinement and/or positive resection margins [35–37]. However, such findings can only be pathologically confirmed by radical prostatectomy. Thus, surgery enables a better selection of patients likely to profit from combined therapy.

The consequences of radical prostatectomy in a locally advanced stage may differ in several respects from those in localized stages.

Continence

In the localized stage and particularly in capsule-confined cancer, maximal sphincter preservation can be achieved by subtle dissection. Continence results are excellent nowadays, as described above [33]. Wide excision prostatectomy is recommended in cases with an increased risk of locally advanced disease. This is not a nerve-sparing procedure. According to recent studies, the finest nerve plexuses associated with continence also run through the pelvic floor region and also near the neurovascular bundles responsible for potency [38, 39]. Thus, the wide excision technique basically harbors a higher risk of postoperative incontinence. Despite these adverse preoperative conditions, the average functional outcomes, though still poorer than in the localized stage, are such that younger patients likewise achieve excellent continence results.

Erectile Dysfunction

As described above, the treatment goal in the locally advanced stage is to achieve negative margins by extending the resection. In the case of a clinically or pathologically non-organ-confined tumor, this may mean removing the neurovascular bundles on 1 or both sides. However, the patient only becomes aware of the clinical consequences of this procedure if there are no (lymph node) metastases. Most patients who have metastases receive long-term hormone withdrawal therapy. The resultant loss of libido lessens the subjective importance the patient attaches to the problem of erectile dysfunction.

As in the localized stage, the results in cases with negative resection margins depend on the preoperative erection status, the patient's age and the preservation of 1 or both neurovascular bundles [33].

Neoadjuvant Therapy

In the course of decades, various studies have examined neoadjuvant therapies before radical prostatectomy to improve its outcome in cases of locally advanced or high-risk cancer. Neoadjuvant hormone therapy is the type most commonly applied. Large studies over the last 10 years have documented pathological downstaging in 8–34% of cases. However, biochemical freedom from recurrence is hardly influenced by this [41–43].

If the preoperative clinical risk classification overrates the real situation, that is, if the tumor is really in a localized stage, a neoadjuvant therapy additionally worsens the results of a potency-preserving nerve-sparing procedure that must basically be considered technically possible in this situation [44]. Thus, there is no evidence that a benefit is derived from neoadjuvant hormone therapy before radical prostatectomy in the locally advanced stage.

Neoadjuvant Chemotherapy and Neoadjuvant Chemohormonal Therapy

Taxanes, alone or combined with other substances, have proved effective in treating hormone-refractory prostate cancer [45, 46]. This supports their preoperative application for neoadjuvant therapy in high-risk cases. If they achieve more effective downstaging than neoadjuvant hormone therapy, it may be possible to improve the results, particularly as regards cancer-specific survival, while avoiding the side effects of hormone therapy. Unfortunately, there have not yet been any large studies to confirm this.

Summing up, it may be said that, even as a monotherapy, radical prostatectomy in the locally advanced stage can achieve a cancer-specific survival of at least 50% after 10 years.

By pathological analysis of the stage, grade and resection margins, the probability of recurrence can be predicted much more precisely with than without surgery. This enables optimal selection and stratification of candidates for adjuvant therapy. Neoadjuvant hormone therapy does not improve functional results or cancer-specific survival.

Conclusion

Radical prostatectomy is the oldest of all treatment modalities for prostate cancer, and its superiority to all other approaches is still impressively documented in the 21st century. This is especially true for younger men, whose long life expectancy lends particular importance to the long follow-up times of the procedure. Functional results (continence and potency preservation) are excellent nowadays, and the complication rate (particularly the transfusion risk) is very low. Precise pathological analysis of the specimen enables more accurate prediction of the prognosis and biochemical recurrence in all tumor stages. Stratified adjuvant therapies or early relapse management can thus be performed. In the locally advanced stage, the overall prognosis is significantly better than with a nonstratified monotherapy. Finally, a particular advantage of radical prostatectomy compared to other treatment modalities is the achievement of postoperative PSA negativity in most cases. This enables the earliest possible detection of a biochemical recurrence.

References

1 Bertz J, Hentschel S, Hundsdörfer G, Kaatsch P, Katalinic A, Lehnert M, Schön D, Stegmaier C, Ziegler H: Krebs in Deutschland, 5. überarbeitete, aktualisierte Ausgabe. Saarbrücken, Gesellschaft der epidemiologischen Krebsregister in Deutschland e.V. und das RKI, 2006.

2 Billroth T: Carcinoma der Prostata, Chir. Erfahrungen. Arch Klin Chir 1869;10:548.

3 Young HH: The cure of cancer of the prostate by radical perineal prostatectomy (prostate-seminal-vesiculectomy). J Urol 1945;53:188–256.

4 Young HH: The early diagnosis and radical cure of carcinoma of the prostate. Being a study of 40 cases and presentation of a radical operation which was carried out in four cases. 1905. J Urol 2002;167:939–946; discussion 947.

5 Pound CR, Brawer MK, Partin AW: Evaluation and treatment of men with biochemical prostate-specific antigen recurrence following definitive therapy for clinically localized prostate cancer. Rev Urol 2001;3:72–84.

6 Lerner SE, Blute ML, Zincke H: Risk factors for progression in patients with prostate cancer treated with radical prostatectomy. Semin Urol Oncol 1996;14:12–20; discussion 21.

7 Stephenson AJ, Scardino PT, Eastham JA, Bianco FJ Jr, Dotan ZA, Fearn PA, Kattan MW: Preoperative nomogram predicting the 10-year probability of prostate cancer recurrence after radical prostatectomy. J Natl Cancer Inst 2006;98:715–717.

8 Karakiewicz PI, Eastham JA, Graefen M, Cagiannos I, Stricker PD, Klein E, Cangiano T, Schroder FH, Scardino PT, Kattan MW: Prognostic impact of positive surgical margins in surgically treated prostate cancer: multi-institutional assessment of 5,831 patients. Urology 2005;66: 1245–1250.

9 Obek C, Lai S, Sadek S, Civantos F, Soloway MS: Age as a prognostic factor for disease recurrence after radical prostatectomy. Urology 1999;54: 533–538.

10 Khan MA, Han M, Partin AW, Epstein JI, Walsh PC: Long-term cancer control of radical prostatectomy in men younger than 50 years of age: update 2003. Urology 2003;62:86–91; discussion 91–92.

11 Khan MA, Partin AW, Mangold LA, Epstein JI, Walsh PC: Probability of biochemical recurrence by analysis of pathologic stage, Gleason score, and margin status for localized prostate cancer. Urology 2003;62:866–871.

12 Freedland SJ, Presti JC Jr, Amling CL, Kane CJ, Aronson WJ, Dorey F, Terris MK: Time trends in biochemical recurrence after radical prostatectomy: results of the SEARCH database. Urology 2003;61:736–741.

13 Moul JW, Connelly RR, Lubeck DP, Bauer JJ, Sun L, Flanders SC, Grossfeld GD, Carroll PR: Predicting risk of prostate specific antigen recurrence after radical prostatectomy with the Center for Prostate Disease Research and Cancer of the Prostate Strategic Urologic Research Endeavor databases. J Urol 2001;166:1322–1327.

14 Graefen M, Noldus J, Pichlmeier U, Haese A, Hammerer P, Fernandez S, Conrad S, Henke R, Huland E, Huland H: Early prostate-specific antigen relapse after radical retropubic prostatectomy: prediction on the basis of preoperative and postoperative tumor characteristics. Eur Urol 1999;36:21–30.

15 Grossfeld GD, Chang JJ, Broering JM, Miller DP, Yu J, Flanders SC, Carroll PR: Does the completeness of prostate sampling predict outcome for patients undergoing radical prostatectomy? Data from the CAPSURE database. Urology 2000;56: 430–435.

16 Han M, Partin AW, Pound CR, Epstein JI, Walsh PC: Long-term biochemical disease-free and cancer-specific survival following anatomic radical retropubic prostatectomy: the 15-year Johns Hopkins experience. Urol Clin North Am 2001; 28:555–565.

17 Aus G, Abbou CC, Bolla M, Heidenreich A, Schmid HP, van Poppel H, Wolff J, Zattoni F: EAU guidelines on prostate cancer. Eur Urol 2005;48:546–551.

18 Catalona WJ, Carvalhal GF, Mager DE, Smith DS: Potency, continence and complication rates in 1,870 consecutive radical retropubic prostatectomies. J Urol 1999;162:433–438.

19 Graefen M, Walz J, Huland H: Open retropubic nerve-sparing radical prostatectomy. Eur Urol 2006;49:38–48.

20 Partin AW, Mangold LA, Lamm DM, Walsh PC, Epstein JI, Pearson JD: Contemporary update of prostate cancer staging nomograms (Partin Tables) for the new millennium. Urology 2001;58: 843–848.

21 Heidenreich A: Intraoperative frozen section analysis to monitor nerve-sparing radical prostatectomy. Eur Urol 2006;49:948–949.

22 Eichelberg C, Erbersdobler A, Haese A, Schlomm T, Chun FK, Currlin E, Walz J, Steuber T, Graefen M, Huland H: Frozen section for the management of intraoperatively detected palpable tumor lesions during nerve-sparing scheduled radical prostatectomy. Eur Urol 2006;49:1011–1016; discussion 1016–1018.

23 Dubbelman YD, Dohle GR, Schroder FH: Sexual function before and after radical retropubic prostatectomy: a systematic review of prognostic indicators for a successful outcome. Eur Urol 2006; 50:711–718; discussion 718–720.

24 Gontero P, Kirby RS: Nerve-sparing radical retropubic prostatectomy: techniques and clinical considerations. Prostate Cancer Prostatic Dis 2005;8:133–139.

25 Gontero P, Kirby R: Proerectile pharmacological prophylaxis following nerve-sparing radical prostatectomy (NSRP). Prostate Cancer Prostatic Dis 2004;7:223–226.

26 Briganti A, Salonia A, Gallina A, Chun FK, Karakiewicz PI, Graefen M, Huland H, Rigatti P, Montorsi F: Management of erectile dysfunction after radical prostatectomy in 2007. World J Urol 2007; 25:143–148.

27 Chang SS, Duong DT, Wells N, Cole EE, Smith JA Jr, Cookson MS: Predicting blood loss and transfusion requirements during radical prostatectomy: the significant negative impact of increasing body mass index. J Urol 2004;171:1861–1865.

28 Friederich PW, Henny CP, Messelink EJ, Geerdink MG, Keller T, Kurth KH, Buller HR, Levi M: Effect of recombinant activated factor VII on perioperative blood loss in patients undergoing retropubic prostatectomy: a double-blind placebo-controlled randomised trial. Lancet 2003;361:201–205.

29 Schwartz K, Bunner S, Bearer R, Severson RK: Complications from treatment for prostate carcinoma among men in the Detroit area. Cancer 2002;95:82–89.

30 Williams D, McCarthy R: Recombinant activated factor VII and perioperative blood loss. Lancet 2003; 361:1745; author reply 1745–1746.

31 Schostak M, Matischak K, Muller M, Schafer M, Schrader M, Christoph F, Miller K: New perioperative management reduces bleeding in radical retropubic prostatectomy. BJU Int 2005;96:316–319.

32 Trabulsi EJ, Guillonneau B: Laparoscopic radical prostatectomy. J Urol 2005;173:1072–1079.

33 Loeb S, Smith ND, Roehl KA, Catalona WJ: Intermediate-term potency, continence, and survival outcomes of radical prostatectomy for clinically high-risk or locally advanced prostate cancer. Urology 2007;69:1170–1175.

34 Hakenberg OW, Frohner M, Wirth MP: Treatment of locally advanced prostate cancer – the case for radical prostatectomy. Urol Int 2006;77: 193–199.

35 Glode LM: The case for adjuvant therapy for prostate cancer. J Urol 2006;176:S30–S33.

36 Skinner EC, Glode LM: High-risk localized prostate cancer: primary surgery and adjuvant therapy. Urol Oncol 2003;21:219–227.

37 Bottke D, Wiegel T: Prevention of local recurrence using adjuvant radiotherapy after radical prostatectomy. Indications, results, and side effects (in German). Urologe A 2006;45:1251–1254.

38 Takenaka A, Tewari AK, Leung RA, Bigelow K, El-Tabey N, Murakami G, Fujisawa M: Preservation of the puboprostatic collar and puboperineoplasty for early recovery of urinary continence after robotic prostatectomy: anatomic basis and preliminary outcomes. Eur Urol 2007; 51:433–440; discussion 440.

39 Takenaka A, Hara R, Soga H, Murakami G, Fujisawa M: A novel technique for approaching the endopelvic fascia in retropubic radical prostatectomy, based on an anatomical study of fixed and fresh cadavers. BJU Int 2005;95: 766–771.

40 D'Amico AV, Hui-Chen M, Renshaw AA, Sussman B, Roehl KA, Catalona WJ: Identifying men diagnosed with clinically localized prostate cancer who are at high risk for death from prostate cancer. J Urol 2006;176:S11–S15.

41 Kumar S, Shelley M, Harrison C, Coles B, Wilt TJ, Mason MD: Neo-adjuvant and adjuvant hormone therapy for localised and locally advanced prostate cancer. Cochrane Database Syst Rev 2006, CD006019.

42 Schulman CC, Debruyne FM, Forster G, Selvaggi FP, Zlotta AR, Witjes WP: 4-year follow-up results of a European prospective randomized study on neoadjuvant hormonal therapy prior to radical prostatectomy in T2-3N0M0 prostate cancer. European Study Group on Neoadjuvant Treatment of Prostate Cancer. Eur Urol 2000;38: 706–713.

43 Civantos F, Sadek S, Obek C, Lai S, Soloway M: Neoadjuvant hormonal therapy prior to radical prostatectomy. Mol Urol 1999;3:201–204.

44 Mantz CA, Nautiyal J, Awan A, Kopnick M, Ray P, Kandel G, Niederberger C, Ignacio L, Dawson E, Fields R, et al: Potency preservation following conformal radiotherapy for localized prostate cancer: impact of neoadjuvant androgen blockade, treatment technique, and patient-related factors. Cancer J Sci Am 1999;5:230–236.

45 Petrylak DP, Tangen CM, Hussain MH, Lara PN Jr, Jones JA, Taplin ME, Burch PA, Berry D, Moinpour C, Kohli M, et al: Docetaxel and estramustine compared with mitoxantrone and prednisone for advanced refractory prostate cancer. N Engl J Med 2004;351:1513–1520.

46 Tannock IF, de Wit R, Berry WR, Horti J, Pluzanska A, Chi KN, Oudard S, Theodore C, James ND, Turesson I, et al: Docetaxel plus prednisone or mitoxantrone plus prednisone for advanced prostate cancer. N Engl J Med 2004;351:1502–1512.

PD Dr. M. Schostak
Department of Urology, Charité Universitätsmedizin Berlin, Campus Benjamin Franklin
Hindenburgdamm 30
DE–12200 Berlin (Germany)
Tel. +49 30 8445 2577, Fax +49 30 8445 4620, E-Mail martin.schostak@charite.de

Moser L, Schostak M, Miller K, Hinkelbein W (eds): Controversies in the Treatment of
Prostate Cancer. Front Radiat Ther Oncol. Basel, Karger, 2008, vol 41, pp 15–25

Radiotherapy as Primary Treatment Modality

M. Sia   T. Rosewall   P. Warde

Department of Radiation Oncology, University of Toronto, and Radiation Medicine Program,
Princess Margaret Hospital, Toronto, Ont., Canada

Abstract

The proper management of prostate cancer is dependent on appropriate risk categorization, based on pretreatment prostate-specific antigen (PSA), clinical stage and Gleason score (GS). The use of radiotherapy in low-risk (T1–T2a, PSA <10 ng/ml and GS ≤6) and intermediate-risk (T1/T2, PSA <20 ng/ml and GS ≤7) disease is well established, with comparable results to surgery in the era of modern radiation therapy. However, cancer-related outcomes in some radiotherapy patients might still be improved with the use of adjuvant hormonal therapy. There is presently no clear evidence to support its use in low-risk patients and benefits in intermediate-risk patients need to be elucidated in the era of dose-escalated radiation therapy. Hypofractionated radiotherapy using biologically equivalent doses also has the potential to improve the therapeutic index, given the low α/β ratio of prostate cancer, and to reduce overall treatment time, but the most advantageous regimen needs to be determined. In patients with high-risk disease (T3–T4, PSA >20 ng/ml or GS ≥8), radiation with hormones has become the standard treatment. The issues that remain focus on determining the optimal duration of hormones, assessing the use of locoregional dose escalation and determining the possible benefit from adjuvant chemotherapy.

In the modern era, >90% of patients present with clinically localized disease and >80% of these fall into the subsets of low- and intermediate-risk disease [1]. Treatment strategies for low- and intermediate-risk prostate cancer include watchful waiting, hormone therapy (for example, androgen deprivation, AD), radical prostatectomy, brachytherapy and external beam radiotherapy (EBRT). The major controversy in the management of low-risk patients is the definition of which patients, if any, benefit from local treatment. Other issues include the choice of local treatment modality, defining the roles of adjunctive hormonal therapy if radia-

Table 1. Risk categories

Risk group	PSA, ng/ml	GS	UICC T stage
Low (all of)	≤10	≤6	≤T2a
Intermediate (any of, if not low risk)	≤20	7	T1/T2
High (any of)	>20	≥8	≥T3

tion therapy is used, radiation dose escalation and fractionation. Based on the data from high-risk disease, the use of neoadjuvant and adjuvant hormonal therapy in patients treated with EBRT has risen substantially over the past decade despite the toxicity of this strategy and the lack of proven clinical benefit. High-risk disease is now routinely approached with combined hormonal therapy and radiotherapy (RT) based on randomized studies that have shown improvements in overall survival [2, 3]. Current issues in the management of these patients include the duration of hormone therapy, the role of adjuvant chemotherapy and the role of dose-escalated EBRT to the primary tumor and the pelvic lymph nodes.

In this manuscript, we will discuss risk categorization in localized prostate cancer and review the controversies in management of localized prostate cancer with particular emphasis on the clinical areas of uncertainty when EBRT is used as the primary treatment modality.

Risk Categorization

Risk stratification systems serve many purposes. Primarily, they are used to accurately correlate the probability of treatment failure and facilitate the selection of the optimal therapeutic approach, but they are also helpful in ensuring prognostic uniformity in clinical trials and in the evaluation of treatment outcomes. The UICC/AJCC TNM staging system is the most widely used system, but fails to incorporate 2 important prognostic factors: pretreatment prostate-specific antigen (PSA) level and Gleason score (GS).

Based on work by D'Amico et al. [4], the Genitourinary Radiation Oncologists of Canada (GUROC) have developed a classification system for patients with localized/locally advanced disease (table 1) [5]. Low-risk prostate cancer is defined as the presence of all of these factors: clinical stage T1–T2a, PSA <10 ng/ml and GS ≤6. High-risk disease is defined as the presence of any of these factors: cT3 or cT4 category, PSA >20 ng/ml or GS ≥8. The intermediate-risk grouping includes all other cases of localized disease. This model has recently been demonstrated to be internally consistent and to accurately predict prostate cancer-specific mortality in patients treated with surgery or radiation therapy [6, 7].

The increased use of PSA screening in the United States over the last 15 years has resulted in a stage migration as evidenced by recent data from the Cancer of the Prostate Strategic Urological Research Endeavor (CaPSURE) registry [1]. The proportion of patients presenting with low-risk disease increased from 31 to 47% between 1989 and 2002, and those presenting with intermediate-risk disease increased from 34 to 37%. In total, more than 80% of all new prostate cancer patients present with low- or intermediate-risk disease and less than 20% present with high-risk tumors.

Low-Risk Disease

PSA-based prostate cancer screening results in the diagnosis of low-risk prostate cancer in many men who are not destined to have clinical progression during their lifetime. In most of these patients, the disease is indolent and slow growing. The challenge to physicians managing these patients is to identify those who are unlikely to experience significant progression, while offering radical therapy to those who are at risk of progressive disease [8]. The National Cancer Institute of Canada Clinical Trials Group (NCIC-CTG) is planning to open a large intergroup trial in 2007 to address the question of whether immediate therapy (surgery or RT) or an approach of close monitoring of patients (active surveillance) with selective delayed intervention based on PSA doubling time should be used to address this important issue (START Trial). Surgeons and radiation oncologists have debated the respective roles of EBRT, radical prostatectomy and interstitial brachytherapy for many years. A recent large multi-institutional study showed equivalent results with all 3 strategies when dose-escalated EBRT was used [9]. It is unlikely that any level 1 evidence will ever be obtained to determine which approach is better (if any). Most practitioners have fixed views on which approach is superior and in addition there are considerable problems in randomizing patients in clinical trials involving different treatment modalities [10].

Adjunctive AD with EBRT in low-risk patients has been discussed at a number of consensus conferences and it is clear that there is no role for the routine use of hormonal therapy [5, 11, 12]. Therefore, the increasing use of EBRT with neoadjuvant hormonal therapy in up to 57% of patients with low-risk disease treated in community practice in the United States is alarming [13]. Unless a subpopulation of low-risk patients with a poor prognosis can be identified, it is unlikely that meaningful results addressing hormonal and radiation therapy will be found, even in the setting of a clinical trial.

Table 2. Benefit of adjunctive hormones in high-risk disease – summary of studies

Study	RTOG 85-31	RTOG 86-10	EORTC 22863	RTOG 92-02	TROG 96-01	
Hormonal therapy duration	indefinite	4 months (neoadjuvant and concurrent)	3 years	2 years	3 months	6 months
Overall survival	15% (10 years)	–	16% (5 years)	–	–	–
Overall survival GS 8–10	17%	–	11%		–	–
Distant metastasis free	10%	11%	19%	5.5%	–	6%
Local control	14%	12%	14%	6%	11%	16%
bNED	24%	14%	31%	27%	14%	16%

bNED = Biochemical freedom from disease.

Intermediate-Risk Disease

Patients with intermediate-risk disease are candidates for surgery or radical radiotherapy. When comparisons are made between the reported studies of radiation and surgery (all retrospective), both treatments appear to be equally effective in terms of local control and survival [9]. The decision to employ radiation rather than surgery is usually made on the basis of patient factors such as age, and the presence of comorbid conditions.

The benefit of dose-escalated radiation therapy has been established in 2 randomized phase III trials and doses ≥ 74 Gy (in 2-Gy fractions) are now routinely used in the management of these patients [14, 15]. The role of adjunctive hormonal therapy is more controversial.

The randomized trial data presented in table 2 show that improvement in local control and/or disease-free or overall survival can be achieved when AD is combined with conventional-dose EBRT in patients with high-risk disease [2, 3, 16–18]. These data are frequently used to justify the use of adjunctive hormonal therapy in patients with intermediate-risk disease. There have been 3 trials assessing the value of hormonal therapy in patients with intermediate risk disease. D'Amico et al. [19] have reported improved overall survival in 206 patients treated at Harvard with EBRT to a dose of 70 Gy and 6 months of AD versus 70 Gy alone (88 vs. 78%, p < 0.04). Approximately 80% of these patients had intermediate-risk disease. Concerns have been raised about this trial including the fact that the difference in survival was based on only 6 prostate cancer-specific deaths in the control arm, with no prostate cancer-specific deaths seen in the experimental arm [20]. Data on the primary study endpoint, biochemical progression, were also not provided in the article. A small study by Laverdiere et al. [21] showed improved PSA-based outcomes using EBRT to a dose of 64 Gy with AD. In this randomized control trial, 70% of patients could be classified as intermediate risk. Further follow-up is necessary to fully evaluate this trial with respect to cancer-related outcomes. In another study, Denham et al. [17] randomly allocated 818 prostate cancer patients to EBRT alone, 3 months of neoadjuvant hormonal therapy or 6 months of neoadjuvant hormonal therapy. There was no difference in overall survival between the arms of the study at a median follow-up of 5.9 years. Patients given neoadjuvant hormonal therapy had better local control of their disease and improved biochemical failure-free survival. Furthermore, patients who received 6 months compared with 3 months of neoadjuvant hormonal treatment had a statistically significant improvement in distant disease failure.

The applicability of the results from these recent studies assessing AD in the intermediate-risk population is complicated by 2 main issues. The first issue is that the randomized control trials showing a benefit of neoadjuvant or adjuvant AD combined with EBRT have largely been completed in patients with high-risk disease. Thus, the conclusions may not be applicable to any or all intermediate-risk patients. The second issue is that the patients in these trials received conventional-dose EBRT (doses <74 Gy). Long-term biochemical freedom from disease rates with EBRT alone using these dose fractionation schemes were poor, approximately 40% in intermediate-risk patients [22–24]. In the Trans-Tasman study group study reported by Denham et al. [17], the radiation dose used was only 66 Gy in 33 fractions over 6.5 weeks – considerably less than currently used in clinical practice.

While there is a lack of level 1 evidence for AD with dose-escalated EBRT for intermediate-risk patients, there are data regarding clinical outcomes from non-randomized, single-institution series in this population of patients. Cavanaugh et al. [25] analyzed a cohort of 1,041 consecutively treated patients with T1–T2 prostate cancer treated with radical prostatectomy, EBRT, brachytherapy (permanent seed implantation) or combined brachytherapy and EBRT. Seven hundred and eighty five patients received EBRT (484 received ≤72 Gy, 301 received >72 Gy) and 143 of these patients were given neoadjuvant AD (≤6 months duration). AD was a significant predictor of biochemical outcome on univariate analysis for the whole patient cohort, but was not significant (p = 0.91) when the group of patients treated to ≤72 Gy was excluded. In another study performed at the Memorial Sloan Kettering Cancer Center, a cohort of 772 patients (89% T1–T2 disease) treated with intensity-modulated radiotherapy (IMRT) to a median dose of 81 Gy demonstrated that AD had no influence on the biochemical freedom from disease at a median follow-up of 24 months [26]. In addition, a large retrospective review of 1,260 patients conducted by Martinez et al. [27] showed a lack of benefit (and a possible detrimental effect) of short-course AD on 5-year metastasis-free survival and cause-specific survival. However, these patients were treated with accelerated hypofractionated pelvic EBRT integrated with transrectal ultrasound-guided conformally modulated high-dose rate brachytherapy. While there is a paucity of definitive evidence from these studies as to the benefit of AD, the role of hormonal therapy in intermediate-risk patients remains unclear and serves to suggest that the addition of AD to dose-escalated EBRT may not be required to optimize biochemical outcome for these patients. The trials by D'Amico et al. [19], Denham et al. [17] and Laverdiere et al. [21] provide some insight into this dilemma, but data using survival endpoints in a true intermediate-risk group of patients treated with AD and dose-escalated EBRT are required. A number of clinical trials are under way to address the role of adjunctive hormonal therapy in these patients, including the 99–07 study at Princess Margaret Hospital in Toronto in which intermediate-risk patients are randomized to either EBRT alone (79.8 Gy in 42 fractions) or EBRT with 5 months of neoadjuvant and concurrent hormonal therapy.

There is some recent evidence that shows that prostate carcinoma does not behave like other carcinomas in terms of responsiveness to radiation therapy. The sensitivity of tissue to radiation fraction size is described by the α- and β-component of the linear quadratic equation [28]. Most carcinomas, and all rapidly dividing normal tissues (acute-reacting tissues), have an α/β ratio of approximately 10 Gy. Slowly dividing late-reacting normal tissues (for example, late fibrosis effect) have an α/β ratio of 3–5 Gy. A number of studies, however, suggest that the α/β ratio for prostate cancer is 0.9–1.5 Gy [29]. The outcome of the only randomized trial of hypofractionated versus conventional prostate RT has suggested that the α/β ratio for prostate cancer is 0.9 [24]. A low α/β ratio for prostate carcinoma suggests that hypofractionated RT might be more efficient at tumor killing than standard fractionation, and could produce equivalent tumor control with a lower total dose and a shorter overall treatment time. This concept is being tested in 2 current clinical trials, one being conducted by the NCIC-CTG and the other by the Radiation Therapy Oncology Group (RTOG) [30].

High-Risk Disease

In the modern era, 15–20% of patients with localized disease fall into the subset of high-risk disease. In the past, the term locally advanced prostate cancer (clinical stage T3–T4) was used to describe these patients, but within the past decade the term high-risk prostate cancer has been coined to encompass this group of patients along with patients with T1/T2 disease with poor prognostic features (either a high PSA or high GS). High-risk prostate cancer is an aggressive disease with poor prognosis as well as significant morbidity and mortality. In 1 study, close to

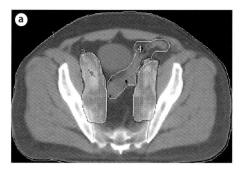 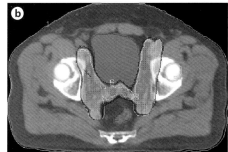

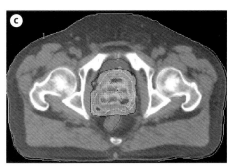

Fig. 1. Three axial computed tomography slices to demonstrate the use of IMRT to conform the color wash of the high isodose region to the clinical target volume for high-risk disease (pelvic lymph nodes, seminal vesicles and prostate). Considerable sparing of the small bowel (**a**), the bladder and rectum (**b**) and the femoral heads (**c**) is possible.

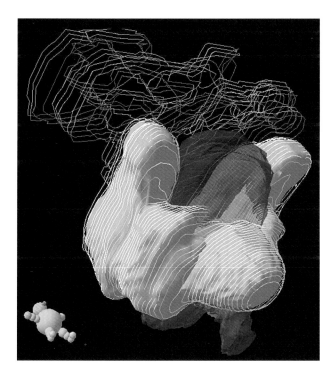

Fig. 2. A three-dimensional model to demonstrate the use of IMRT to conform the isodoses (white wireframe) to the complex shape of the high-risk clinical target volume (blue solid), while avoiding the small bowel (blue wireframe), bladder and rectum (pink solid).

50% of men with high-risk tumors died of prostate cancer within 10 years of diagnosis, compared with 6% and 0% of patients with intermediate- and low-risk disease, respectively [7].

Radiation therapy has been the mainstay of treatment in the management of patients with high-risk disease for the past 30 years. However, results with RT alone have been poor and multiple studies have demonstrated the benefit of adjunctive hormonal therapy [2, 3]. The benefit of local therapy in this disease is unclear, as many patients are felt to harbor subclinical metastases at presentation. Similar outcomes in terms of overall survival to those seen with RT alone have been reported with hormonal therapy alone [31, 32]. The NCI-CTG/MRC PR-3 phase III randomized trial has been recently completed (1,205 patients) and is powered to detect a small benefit in overall survival from the addition of RT to primary hormonal therapy [33]. This trial, in addition to assessing the benefit of RT on overall survival, will assess the impact of locoregional RT on symptomatic local control of disease and quality of life.

The optimal duration of adjuvant hormonal therapy is unclear. The RTOG 92–02 study randomized 1,554 patients to 4 or 28 months of hormonal therapy and, on preliminary subset analysis, there was an overall survival benefit (81 vs. 70.7%, p = 0.044) seen with the use of prolonged hormonal therapy in patients with GS 8–10 tumors [16]. The EORTC 22961 trial comparing 6 versus 36 months of adjuvant RT accrued 966 patients and closed in May 2002. This trial, along with mature results from the RTOG 92–02 study should establish whether prolonged adjuvant hormonal therapy is necessary in this setting.

As discussed earlier, in patients with low- and intermediate-risk disease there is now clear evidence from phase III randomized trials that RT dose escalation using three-dimensional conformal RT or IMRT improves biochemical freedom from disease outcomes. While there are no randomized trials of dose escalation in high-risk disease, various institutional retrospective studies have suggested that dose escalation in this subgroup of patients may also have substantial benefits [34, 35]. Patients with high-risk prostate cancer have a moderate to high risk of occult lymph node-metastatic disease. There is some evidence to suggest that prophylactic nodal irradiation using conventional-dose RT improves progression-free survival, while other trials have produced negative results [36, 37]. Using IMRT, it is now possible to perform dose escalation to the pelvic lymph nodes with minimal acute bladder and small bowel toxicity [38]. A typical dose distribution is shown in figure 1, demonstrating that the bladder and adjacent small bowel can be kept out of the high-dose area. A wire frame rendering of an IMRT dose distribution for prostate and pelvic nodes of a recent case treated at the Princess Margaret Hospital is shown in figure 2. The long-term efficacy and toxicity of this approach is not known and randomized clinical trials are necessary to evaluate this strategy.

Recent data showing improved survival in patients with hormone-refractory prostate cancer treated with docetaxel-containing regimens have raised the possibility that adjuvant chemotherapy might be effective in patients with localized disease [39, 40]. An NCIC-CTG randomized phase III study comparing EBRT and hormonal therapy with or without neoadjuvant docetaxel is currently accruing patients and a similar study is also being conducted by the RTOG (using adjuvant docetaxel).

Conclusions

In low-risk prostate cancer the most important issue to resolve over the next decade is to define which patients benefit from local therapy. In intermediate-risk disease the key issues (in terms of EBRT) are to determine the role of adjunctive hormonal therapy and the best dose fractionation scheme. In high-risk disease, adjunctive chemotherapy and radiation dose escalation both hold out the promise of significant benefit and need to be evaluated. Only by accruing patients to prospective randomized trials will all these issues be addressed.

References

1 Cooperberg MR, Lubeck DP, Mehta SS, Carroll PR: Time trends in clinical risk stratification for prostate cancer: implications for outcomes (data from CaPSURE). J Urol 2003;170:S21–S25; discussion S26–S27.

2 Pilepich MV, Winter K, Lawton CA, Krisch RE, Wolkov HB, Movsas B, Hug EB, Asbell SO, Grignon D: Androgen suppression adjuvant to definitive radiotherapy in prostate carcinoma-long-term results of phase III RTOG 85-31. Int J Radiat Oncol Biol Phys 2005;61:1285–1290.

3 Bolla M, Collette L, Blank L, Warde P, Dubois JB, Mirimanoff RO, Storme G, Bernier J, Kuten A, Sternberg C, Mattelaer J, Lopez Torecilla J, Pfeffer JR, Lino Cutajar C, Zurlo A, Pierart M: Long-term results with immediate androgen suppression and external irradiation in patients with locally advanced prostate cancer (an EORTC study): a phase III randomised trial. Lancet 2002; 360:103–106.

4 D'Amico AV, Desjardin A, Chung A, Chen MH, Schultz D, Whittington R, Malkowicz SB, Wein A, Tomaszewski JE, Renshaw AA, Loughlin K, Richie JP: Assessment of outcome prediction models for patients with localized prostate carcinoma managed with radical prostatectomy or external beam radiation therapy. Cancer 1998;82: 1887–1896.

5 Lukka H, Warde P, Pickles T, Morton G, Brundage M, Souhami L: Controversies in prostate cancer radiotherapy: consensus development. Can J Urol 2001;8:1314–1322.

6 Chism DB, Hanlon AL, Horwitz EM, Feigenberg SJ, Pollack A: A comparison of the single and double factor high-risk models for risk assignment of prostate cancer treated with 3D conformal radiotherapy. Int J Radiat Oncol Biol Phys 2004;59:380–385.

7 D'Amico AV, Cote K, Loffredo M, Renshaw AA, Schultz D: Determinants of prostate cancer specific survival following radiation therapy during the prostate specific antigen era. J Urol 2003;170: S42–S46; discussion S46–S47.

8 Klotz L: Active surveillance for prostate cancer: for whom? J Clin Oncol 2005;23:8165–8169.

9 Kupelian P, Potters L, Khuntia D, Ciezki JP, Reddy C, Reuther AM, Carlson TP, Klein EA: Radical prostatectomy, external beam radiotherapy <72 Gy, external beam radiotherapy > or = 72 Gy, permanent seed implantation, or combined seeds/external beam radiotherapy for stage T1-T2 prostate cancer. Int J Rad Onc Biol Phys 2004;58:25–33.

10 Wallace K, Fleshner N, Jewett M, Basiuk J, Crook J: Impact of a multi-disciplinary patient education session on accrual to a difficult clinical trial: the Toronto experience with the surgical prostatectomy versus interstitial radiation intervention trial. J Clin Oncol 2006;24:4158–4162.

11 Lukka H, Pickles T, Morton G, Catton C, Souhami L, Warde P: Prostate cancer radiotherapy 2002: the way forward. Can J Urol 2005;12:2521–2531.

12 Carroll PR, Kantoff PW, Balk SP, Brown MA, D'Amico AV, George DJ, Grossfeld GD, Johnson CS, Kelly WK, Klotz L, Lee WR, Lubeck DP, McLeod DG, Oh WK, Pollack A, Sartor O, Smith MR, Hart C: Overview consensus statement. Newer approaches to androgen deprivation therapy in prostate cancer. Urology 2002;60(suppl 1):1–6.

13 Cooperberg MR, Grossfeld GD, Lubeck DP, Carroll PR: National practice patterns and time trends in androgen ablation for localized prostate cancer. J Natl Cancer Inst 2003;95:981–989.

14 Zietman AL, DeSilvio ML, Slater JD, Rossi CJ Jr, Miller DW, Adams JA, Shipley WU: Comparison of conventional-dose versus high-dose conformal radiation therapy in clinically localized adenocarcinoma of the prostate: a randomized controlled trial. JAMA 2005;294:1233–1239.

15 Pollack A, Zagars GK, Starkschall G, Antolak JA, Lee JJ, Huang E, von Eschenbach AC, Kuban DA, Rosen I: Prostate cancer radiation dose response: results of the M.D. Anderson phase III randomized trial. Int J Radiat Oncol Biol Phys 2002;53:1097–1105.

16 Hanks GE, Pajak TF, Porter A, Grignon D, Brereton H, Venkatesan V, Horwitz EM, Lawton C, Rosenthal SA, Sandler HM, Shipley WU: Phase III trial of long-term adjuvant androgen deprivation after neoadjuvant hormonal cytoreduction and radiotherapy in locally advanced carcinoma of the prostate: the Radiation Therapy Oncology Group Protocol 92-02. J Clin Oncol 2003;21:3972–3978.

17 Denham JW, Steigler A, Lamb DS, Joseph D, Mameghan H, Turner S, Matthews J, Franklin I, Atkinson C, North J, Poulsen M, Christie D, Spry NA, Tai KH, Wynne C, Duchesne G, Kovacev O, D'Este C: Short-term androgen deprivation and radiotherapy for locally advanced prostate cancer: results from the Trans-Tasman Radiation Oncology Group 96.01 randomised controlled trial. Lancet Oncol 2005;6:841–850.

18 Pilepich MV, Winter K, John MJ, Mesic JB, Sause W, Rubin P, Lawton C, Machtay M, Grignon D: Phase III Radiation Therapy Oncology Group (RTOG) trial 86-10 of androgen deprivation adjuvant to definitive radiotherapy in locally advanced carcinoma of the prostate. Int J Radiat Oncol Biol Phys 2001;50:1243–1252.

19 D'Amico AV, Manola J, Loffredo M, Renshaw AA, DellaCroce A, Kantoff PW: 6-month androgen suppression plus radiation therapy vs radiation therapy alone for patients with clinically localized prostate cancer: a randomized controlled trial. JAMA 2004;292:821–827.

20 DeWeese TL: Radiation therapy and androgen suppression as treatment for clinically localized prostate cancer: the new standard? JAMA 2004;292:864–866.

21 Laverdiere J, Nabid A, De Bedoya LD, Ebacher A, Fortin A, Wang CS, Harel F: The efficacy and sequencing of a short course of androgen suppression on freedom from biochemical failure when administered with radiation therapy for T2–T3 prostate cancer. J Urol 2004;171:1137–1140.

22 Catton C, Gospodarowicz M, Mui J, Panzarella T, Milosevic M, McLean M, Catton P, Warde P: Clinical and biochemical outcome of conventional dose radiotherapy for localized prostate cancer. Can J Urol 2002;9:1444–1452; discussion 1453.

23 Zietman AL, Chung CS, Coen JJ, Shipley WU: 10-year outcome for men with localized prostate cancer treated with external radiation therapy: results of a cohort study. J Urol 2004;171:210–214.

24 Lukka H, Hayter C, Julian JA, Warde P, Morris WJ, Gospodarowicz M, Levine M, Sathya J, Choo R, Prichard H, Brundage M, Kwan W: Randomized trial comparing two fractionation schedules for patients with localized prostate cancer. J Clin Oncol 2005;23:6132–6138.

25 Cavanaugh SX, Kupelian PA, Fuller CD, Reddy C, Bradshaw P, Pollock BH, Fuss M: Early prostate-specific antigen (PSA) kinetics following prostate carcinoma radiotherapy: prognostic value of a time-and-PSA threshold model. Cancer 2004;101:96–105.

26 Zelefsky MJ, Fuks Z, Hunt M, Yamada Y, Marion C, Ling CC, Amols H, Venkatraman ES, Leibel SA: High-dose intensity modulated radiation therapy for prostate cancer: early toxicity and biochemical outcome in 772 patients. Int J Radiat Oncol Biol Phys 2002;53:1111–1116.

27 Martinez AA, Demanes DJ, Galalae R, Vargas C, Bertermann H, Rodriguez R, Gustafson G, Altieri G, Gonzalez J: Lack of benefit from a short course of androgen deprivation for unfavorable prostate cancer patients treated with an accelerated hypofractionated regime. Int J Radiat Oncol Biol Phys 2005;62:1322–1331.

28 Hill RP, Rodemann HP, Hendry JH, Roberts SA, Anscher MS: Normal tissue radiobiology: from the laboratory to the clinic. Int J Radiat Oncol Biol Phys 2001;49:353–365.

29 Fowler JF, Ritter MA, Chappell RJ, Brenner DJ: What hypofractionated protocols should be tested for prostate cancer? Int J Radiat Oncol Biol Phys 2003;56:1093–1104.

30 Lock M, Catton C: High-precision radiotherapy: where are we going and how do we get there? Can J Urol 2006;13(suppl):234–236.

31 Fellows GJ, Clark PB, Beynon LL, Boreham J, Keen C, Parkinson MC, Peto R, Webb JN: Treatment of advanced localised prostatic cancer by orchiectomy, radiotherapy, or combined treatment. A Medical Research Council Study. Urological Cancer Working Party – Subgroup on Prostatic Cancer. Br J Urol 1992;70:304–309.

32 Labrie F, Cusan L, Gomez JL, Belanger A, Candas B: Long-term combined androgen blockade alone for localized prostate cancer. Mol Urol 1999;3:217–226.

33 Mason M, Warde P, Sydes M, Cowan R, James N, Kirkbride P, Langley R, Latham J, Moynihan C, Anderson J, Millet J, Nutall J, Moffat L, Parulekar W, Parmar M: Defining the need for local therapy in locally advanced prostate cancer: an appraisal of the MRC PR07 study. Clin Oncol (R Coll Radiol) 2005;17:217–218.

34 Jacob R, Hanlon AL, Horwitz EM, Movsas B, Uzzo RG, Pollack A: Role of prostate dose escalation in patients with greater than 15% risk of pelvic lymph node involvement. Int J Radiat Oncol Biol Phys 2005;61:695–701.

35 Cheung R, Tucker SL, Dong L, Kuban D: Dose-response for biochemical control among high-risk prostate cancer patients after external beam radiotherapy. Int J Radiat Oncol Biol Phys 2003;56:1234–1240.

36 Asbell SO, Krall JM, Pilepich MV, Baerwald H, Sause WT, Hanks GE, Perez CA: Elective pelvic irradiation in stage A2, B carcinoma of the prostate: analysis of RTOG 77-06. Int J Radiat Oncol Biol Phys 1988;15:1307–1316.

37 Roach M 3rd, DeSilvio M, Valicenti R, Grignon D, Asbell SO, Lawton C, Thomas CR Jr, Shipley WU: Whole-pelvis, 'mini-pelvis', or prostate-only external beam radiotherapy after neoadjuvant and concurrent hormonal therapy in patients treated in the Radiation Therapy Oncology Group 9413 trial. Int J Radiat Oncol Biol Phys 2006;66:647–653.

38 Cavey ML, Bayouth JE, Colman M, Endres EJ, Sanguineti G: IMRT to escalate the dose to the prostate while treating the pelvic nodes. Strahlenther Onkol 2005;181:431–441.

39 Petrylak DP, Tangen CM, Hussain MH, Lara PN Jr, Jones JA, Taplin ME, Burch PA, Berry D, Moinpour C, Kohli M, Benson MC, Small EJ, Raghavan D, Crawford ED: Docetaxel and estramustine compared with mitoxantrone and prednisone for advanced refractory prostate cancer. N Engl J Med 2004;351:1513–1520.

40 Tannock IF, de Wit R, Berry WR, Horti J, Pluzanska A, Chi KN, Oudard S, Theodore C, James ND, Turesson I, Rosenthal MA, Eisenberger MA: Docetaxel plus prednisone or mitoxantrone plus prednisone for advanced prostate cancer. N Engl J Med 2004;351:1502–1512.

Dr. Padraig Warde
Department of Radiation Oncology, Princess Margaret Hospital
610 University Avenue
Toronto, Ont., M5G 2M9 (Canada)
Tel. +1 416 946 2122, Fax +1 416 946 4586, E-Mail padraig.warde@rmp.uhn.on.ca

Moser L, Schostak M, Miller K, Hinkelbein W (eds): Controversies in the Treatment of
Prostate Cancer. Front Radiat Ther Oncol. Basel, Karger, 2008, vol 41, pp 26–31

Combined Radiotherapy and Hormonal Therapy in the Treatment of Prostate Cancer

Dirk Boehmer

Department of Radiation Oncology, Charité Universitätsmedizin Berlin,
Campus Virchow Klinikum, Berlin, Germany

Abstract

The use of hormonal therapy as an adjunct to radiotherapy has been discussed controversially for years. Results of large RTOG and EORTC trials indicate that the combination of these treatment modalities may improve survival in subsets of patients. Many questions with respect to onset, duration, type of hormonal therapy and appropriate patient selection are still under investigation. Following a short overview of the corresponding literature, evidence-based recommendations for daily clinical practice are provided.

Hormonal therapy has been used for decades as the sole treatment or as an adjunct to radiotherapy in patients suffering from prostate cancer. There are numerous drugs that have proven to be efficacious and that have been used in various clinical situations. Table 1 summarizes the most frequently prescribed drugs, including their mechanism of action as well as main side effects.

In the early 1990s the Radiation Therapy Oncology Group (RTOG) conducted a phase II trial (RTOG 85-19) which used an induction hormonal therapy of a luteinizing hormone-releasing hormone (LHRH) agonist together with an anti-androgen before initiation of external beam radiotherapy (EBRT) for patients with bulky prostate cancer [1]. They found encouraging response rates with this combination. Another early study on the possible effects of hormonal therapy was conducted by Zelefsky et al. [2], who performed radiotherapy treatment planning on a group of patients with bulky prostate cancer. After evaluation of dose volume histograms, 22 patients were included in whom more than 30% of

Table 1. Selection of frequently prescribed drugs in hormonal therapy of prostate cancer

Trade name (examples)	Substance	Mechanism	Main side effects
Fugerel Casodex	flutamide bicalutamide	nonsteroidal antiandrogen	flushes, depression, liver toxicity, gynecomastia
Androcur	cyproterone acetate	steroidal antiandrogen	thromboembolic complications, flushes
Estradurin	polyestradiol phosphate	inhibition of LH/FSH-RH	thromboembolic complications, heart attack
Zoladex Enantone Pamorelin	goserelin leuprorelin triptorelin	LHRH agonist	erectile dysfunction, hot flushes, sweating

LH = Luteinizing hormone; FSH = follicle-stimulating hormone; RH = releasing hormone.

the rectal and more than 50% of the bladder volume would receive 95% of the prescription dose.

They received 3 months of an LHRH agonist plus flutamide therapy. Thereafter, the planning procedure was repeated and showed improvements with respect to high irradiation doses in all investigated volumes.

In a similar study of 107 patients, Kucway et al. [3] found that there was a significant correlation between prostate volume reduction and the initial volume as well as the duration of hormonal therapy. Moreover, they found that a maximum androgen blockage using an antiandrogen together with LHRH agonists significantly increased volume reduction compared to LHRH agonist administration alone ($p = 0.04$).

Statement: Hormonal therapy may reduce the prostate volume and thus may also decrease the dose of radiation to volumes of organs at risk such as the rectum or bladder (level of evidence: 3).

The main objective of the combination of radiation and hormonal therapy is the additional effect of androgen deprivation on tumor cell kill or inactivation, respectively. There are various in vitro data about the direct or mediated inhibitory effect of hormonal therapy on prostate cancer cells [4–7]. Nevertheless, we are lacking validated clinical data on the cellular effect of androgen deprivation [8, 9].

The question which risk group would benefit most, whether to apply hormonal therapy in a neoadjuvant, concomitant or in an adjuvant setting, and the duration of hormonal therapy application, have been discussed controversially for years.

Since the mid 1980s, prospective phase III trials have been carried out in order to answer basic questions of the additive effect of hormonal therapy when combined with radiotherapy [2 large trials from the RTOG (trials 85-31 and 86-10) and 1 from the European Organization for Research and Treatment of Cancer (EORTC 22863)] [10–22].

The latter trial evaluated 415 patients with locally advanced prostate cancer with a primary tumor that extended beyond the prostate capsule (T3–T4, 89% of all patients) or organ-confined disease (T1–T2) with unfavorable histology. The overall survival was significantly improved in the combined treatment arm, 78 versus 62% in the radiotherapy only arm. Also, the clinical disease-free survival was significantly improved, 74 versus 40%.

This EORTC trial was the first to demonstrate that there is a significant survival advantage for patients treated with a combination of androgen deprivation therapy and radiotherapy.

In the RTOG 85-31 trial, 977 patients with palpable primary tumor extending beyond the prostate (clinical stage T3) or those with regional lymphatic involvement (T1–2, N+) were randomized to receive either (1) radiotherapy together with goserelin 3.6 mg therapy (every 4 weeks) started during the last week of radiotherapy and continued indefinitely or until signs of disease progression emerged, or (2) radiotherapy alone followed by observation and administration of goserelin at the time of progression. Patients were well matched in relation to Gleason score, lymph node involvement, history of prostatectomy and acid phosphatase.

The authors concluded for 945 evaluable patients that goserelin as an adjuvant to radiotherapy significantly reduced disease progression and improved absolute survival. The treatment was regarded as the standard of care in patients with unfavorable prostate cancer, especially for those with a high Gleason score.

In the RTOG 86-10 trial, 471 patients were randomized either to neoadjuvant and concomitant hormonal therapy plus radiotherapy or to radiotherapy alone. Eligible patients had bulky primary tumors, clinical stage T2–T4, which were defined clinically based on digital rectal examination. Patients with positive lymph nodes were also eligible if the involved nodes remained below the common iliac level. With a median follow-up of 6.7 years for all patients and 8.6 years for patients alive, biochemical no evidence of disease (bNED) was significantly improved with combination therapy ($p = 0.004$), the rate of distant metastases was marginally reduced ($p = 0.04$). A subset analysis indicated that the beneficial effect of hormonal management appears preferentially in patients with lower Gleason score (2–6). In this population, experimental treatment was associated with a highly significant improvement in all endpoints, including survival ($p = 0.015$).

Statement: Short-term hormonal therapy and radiotherapy significantly improve overall survival, distant metastasis-free survival and bNED in intermediate- and high-risk patients with a Gleason score of 2–6 (level of evidence: 1b).

Long-term hormonal therapy and radiotherapy significantly improve overall survival, distant metastasis free-survival and bNED in patients with locally advanced prostate cancer (level of evidence: 1).

Despite these phase III study results, several questions are not answered and remain to be addressed:

(1) What is the optimal timing of androgen deprivation therapy? What is the optimal duration of neoadjuvant hormonal therapy?
(2) What is the optimal overall treatment time of hormonal therapy in intermediate- and high-risk patients?
(3) Which is the optimal androgen deprivation therapy: antiandrogens, LHRH agonists or a combination of both?
(4) Which is the subset of patients who do not benefit from androgen deprivation therapy at all?

The question of duration of neoadjuvant hormonal therapy was addressed by Crook et al. [23] in a phase III trial randomizing 378 patients to either 3 or 8 months of neoadjuvant hormonal treatment. They found no significant improvement in tumor-specific or overall survival for 1 of the 2 groups [23]. The overall duration of hormonal therapy was investigated in a phase III trial (RTOG 92-02). All patients received hormonal therapy neoadjuvant and concomitant to EBRT. Patients were randomized to either receive a 24-month adjuvant LHRH therapy or not. After a median follow-up of 5.8 years, the hormonal therapy group demonstrated a highly significant advantage in terms of disease-free survival [24].

The role of hormonal therapy was widely evaluated in the early prostate cancer trial (EPC trial), which accrued more than 8,100 patients with prostate cancer. Patients were randomized to receive either placebo or bicalutamide with standard of care (radical prostatectomy, radiotherapy or watchful waiting). The subset analysis of the irradiated patients revealed a significantly reduced risk of disease progression in the bicalutamide arm after a median follow-up of 7.2 years [25].

In conclusion, there is evidence that neoadjuvant hormonal therapy reduces the prostate volume. For low-risk patients (<T2b *and* Gleason score <7 *and* PSA <10), there is (at present) no evidence for an advantage of hormonal therapy combined with EBRT. With respect to high-risk patients, a combination of hormonal therapy and EBRT can be regarded as the standard of care. For intermediate-risk patients, there is no clear recommendation. A short-term hormonal therapy (for example, 6 months) may improve survival in a subset of patients.

References

1 Pilepich MV, John MJ, Krall JM, et al: Phase II Radiation Therapy Oncology Group study of hormonal cytoreduction with flutamide and Zoladex in locally advanced carcinoma of the prostate treated with definitive radiotherapy. Am J Clin Oncol 1990;13:461–464.

2 Zelefsky MJ, Leibel SA, Burman CM, et al: Neoadjuvant hormonal therapy improves the therapeutic ratio in patients with bulky prostatic cancer treated with three-dimensional conformal radiation therapy. Int J Radiat Oncol Biol Phys 1994;29:755–761.

3 Kucway R, Vicini F, Huang R, et al: Prostate volume reduction with androgen deprivation therapy before interstitial brachytherapy. J Urol 2002; 167:2443–2447.

4 Dondi D, Festuccia C, Piccolella M, et al: GnRH agonists and antagonists decrease the metastatic progression of human prostate cancer cell lines by inhibiting the plasminogen activator system. Oncol Rep 2006;15:393–400.

5 Angelucci C, Iacopino F, Lama G, et al: Apoptosis-related gene expression affected by a GnRH analogue without induction of programmed cell death in LNCaP cells. Anticancer Res 2004;24: 2729–2738.

6 Cheng L, Zhang S, Sweeney CJ, et al: Androgen withdrawal inhibits tumor growth and is associated with decrease in angiogenesis and VEGF expression in androgen-independent CWR22Rv1 human prostate cancer model. Anticancer Res 2004;24:2135–2140.

7 Marelli MM, Moretti RM, Dondi D, et al. Luteinizing hormone-releasing hormone agonists interfere with the mitogenic activity of the insulin-like growth factor system in androgen-independent prostate cancer cells. Endocrinology 1999;140:329–334.

8 Polito M, Muzzonigro G, Minardi D, et al. Effects of neoadjuvant androgen deprivation therapy on prostatic cancer. Eur Urol 1996;30(suppl 1):26–31; discussion 38–39.

9 Hintz BL, Koo C, Murphy JF: Pattern of proliferative index (Ki-67) after anti-androgen manipulation reflects the ability of irradiation to control prostate cancer. Am J Clin Oncol 2004;27:85–88.

10 Bolla M, Collette L, Blank L, et al: Long-term results with immediate androgen suppression and external irradiation in patients with locally advanced prostate cancer (an EORTC study): a phase III randomised trial. Lancet 2002;360:103–106.

11 Bolla M, de Reijke TM, Zurlo A, et al: Adjuvant hormone therapy in locally advanced and localized prostate cancer: three EORTC trials. Front Radiat Ther Oncol 2002;36:81–86.

12 Bolla M, Gonzalez D, Warde P, et al: Improved survival in patients with locally advanced prostate cancer treated with radiotherapy and goserelin. N Engl J Med 1997;337:295–300.

13 Corn BW, Winter K, Pilepich MV: Does androgen suppression enhance the efficacy of postoperative irradiation? A secondary analysis of RTOG 85-31. Radiation Therapy Oncology Group. Urology 1999;54:495–502.

14 Horwitz EM, Winter K, Hanks GE, et al: Subset analysis of RTOG 85-31 and 86-10 indicates an advantage for long-term vs. short-term adjuvant hormones for patients with locally advanced nonmetastatic prostate cancer treated with radiation therapy. Int J Radiat Oncol Biol Phys 2001; 49:947–956.

15 Lawton CA, Winter K, Byhardt R, et al: Androgen suppression plus radiation versus radiation alone for patients with D1 (pN+) adenocarcinoma of the prostate (results based on a national prospective randomized trial, RTOG 85-31). Radiation Therapy Oncology Group. Int J Radiat Oncol Biol Phys 1997;38:931–939.

16 Lawton CA, Winter K, Grignon D, et al: Androgen suppression plus radiation versus radiation alone for patients with stage D1/pathologic node-positive adenocarcinoma of the prostate: updated results based on national prospective randomized trial Radiation Therapy Oncology Group 85-31. J Clin Oncol 2005;23:800–807.

17 Lawton CA, Winter K, Murray K, et al: Updated results of the phase III Radiation Therapy Oncology Group (RTOG) trial 85-31 evaluating the potential benefit of androgen suppression following standard radiation therapy for unfavorable prognosis carcinoma of the prostate. Int J Radiat Oncol Biol Phys 2001;49:937–946.

18 Pilepich MV, Caplan R, Byhardt RW, et al: Phase III trial of androgen suppression using goserelin in unfavorable-prognosis carcinoma of the prostate treated with definitive radiotherapy: report of Radiation Therapy Oncology Group Protocol 85-31. J Clin Oncol 1997;15:1013–1021.

19 Pilepich MV, Winter K, John MJ, et al: Phase III radiation therapy oncology group (RTOG) trial 86-10 of androgen deprivation adjuvant to definitive radiotherapy in locally advanced carcinoma of the prostate. Int J Radiat Oncol Biol Phys 2001; 50:1243–1252.

20 Pilepich MV, Winter K, Lawton CA, et al: Androgen suppression adjuvant to definitive radiotherapy in prostate carcinoma – long-term results of phase III RTOG 85-31. Int J Radiat Oncol Biol Phys 2005;61:1285–1290.

21 Shipley WU, Desilvio M, Pilepich MV, et al: Early initiation of salvage hormone therapy influences survival in patients who failed initial radiation for locally advanced prostate cancer: a secondary analysis of RTOG protocol 86-10. Int J Radiat Oncol Biol Phys 2006;64:1162–1167.

22 Shipley WU, Lu JD, Pilepich MV, et al: Effect of a short course of neoadjuvant hormonal therapy on the response to subsequent androgen suppression in prostate cancer patients with relapse after radiotherapy: a secondary analysis of the randomized protocol RTOG 86-10. Int J Radiat Oncol Biol Phys 2002;54:1302–1310.

23 Crook J, Ludgate C, Malone S, et al: Report of a multicenter Canadian phase III randomized trial of 3 months vs. 8 months neoadjuvant androgen deprivation before standard-dose radiotherapy for clinically localized prostate cancer. Int J Radiat Oncol Biol Phys 2004;60:15–23.

24 Hanks GE, Pajak TF, Porter A, et al: Phase III trial of long-term adjuvant androgen deprivation after neoadjuvant hormonal cytoreduction and radiotherapy in locally advanced carcinoma of the prostate: the Radiation Therapy Oncology Group Protocol 92-02. J Clin Oncol 2003;21: 3972–3978.

25 Tyrrell CJ, Payne H, See WA, et al: Bicalutamide ('Casodex') 150 mg as adjuvant to radiotherapy in patients with localised or locally advanced prostate cancer: results from the randomised Early Prostate Cancer Programme. Radiother Oncol 2005;76:4–10.

Dr. Dirk Boehmer
Department of Radiation Oncology, Charité Universitätsmedizin Berlin, Campus Virchow Klinikum
Augustenburger Platz 1
DE–13353 Berlin (Germany)
Tel. +49 30 450 527 052, Fax +49 30 450 527 917, E-Mail dirk.boehmer@charite.de

Moser L, Schostak M, Miller K, Hinkelbein W (eds): Controversies in the Treatment of
Prostate Cancer. Front Radiat Ther Oncol. Basel, Karger, 2008, vol 41, pp 32–38

Postoperative Adjuvant Radiotherapy – Standard of Care?

Dirk Bottke   Thomas Wiegel

Department of Radiotherapy and Radiation Oncology, University Hospital Ulm,
Ulm, Germany

Abstract

Background: Within 5 years following radical prostatectomy, between 15 and 60% of patients with pT3 prostate carcinomas show an increasing prostate-specific antigen (PSA) level as a sign of local and/or systemic tumor progression. Apart from a large number of retrospective investigations, results are available from 3 randomized studies. **Results:** For pT3 prostate carcinomas, the data from the 3 randomized studies agree, showing a reduced biochemical progression rate after 4–5 years of around 20%. The majority of authors use total doses of 60 Gy with single doses of 2 Gy. The rate of severe late side effects is below 2%. The data for pT2 prostate carcinomas with positive margins are worse. Here, controversy exists, and further investigations are required. **Conclusions:** The effectiveness of adjuvant radiotherapy for patients with pT3 tumors with positive margins with and without undetectable PSA levels is proposed. However, a survival advantage has not been demonstrated to date. For patients with positive margins in organ-limited prostate carcinomas (pT2 R1), randomized studies are recommended. It is unclear whether adjuvant radiotherapy is superior to radiotherapy for PSA levels rising out of the undetectable range after radical prostatectomy.

Postprostatectomy examination of clinically staged T1/2 adenocarcinomas of the prostate reveal a T3/4 pathologic stage in up to 25% of cases; this probability increases to over 40% in clinical T2b tumors [1–3]. Radical prostatectomy is also frequently performed in patients with clinical stage T3 carcinomas. In these patients, the probability of postoperative tumor growth beyond the organ is 80%. In approximately 20% of cases this is clinical overstaging [4]. The positive margin after radical prostatectomy is of substantial prognostic importance [5]. While it is rare in stage pT2, it is common for pT3 tumors also in hospitals with high surgical volume. The absolute numbers for this amount to 5–10% of R1 resections in tumor stage pT2 and 10–40% in stage pT3; in large centers up to 25% of R1 resections for pT3 carcinomas are not unusual [1].

While the meaning of the positive margins is debated in tumor stage pT2, it is indisputable that in tumor stage pT3 positive margins represent an independent risk for biochemical progression [5–7]. With regard to this positive margin, it seems reasonable to suppose remaining microscopic tumor usually obvious at the height of the anastomosis region, but also in the resection bed of the prostate. This remaining microscopic tumor represents the target volume of the adjuvant percutaneous three-dimensional planned radiotherapy (RT), which is usually performed with 60 Gy over 6 weeks. The majority of authors see reaching the PSA undetectable range as a condition for the definition 'adjuvant RT', the definition of this range, however, is very different (between <0.1 and <0.03 ng/ml). Up to 60% of patients defined in such a way exhibit an increase in prostate-specific antigen (PSA) from the undetectable range within 5 years, usually without clinically provable correlate [3]. On the other hand, it is well known that in 35–54% of the patients with rising PSA after radical prostatectomy without clinically correlate, vital tumor tissue was found only by punch biopsies from the urethrovesical anastomosis [8]. These results support the use of adjuvant RT after radical prostatectomy. The proceeding of urologists with patients with positive margins, in particular in stage pT2 R1, but also in stage pT3 R1, is controversial. Different authors suggest 'watchful waiting', delayed or immediate hormone therapy, or adjuvant RT or RT only in case of rising PSA [9–13]. Adjuvant RT became more attractive after the introduction of three-dimensional treatment planning as well as intensity-modulated RT, thus reducing acute and late side effects [14]. This overview examines the results and possible therapy sequences for patients after radical prostatectomy with or without positive margins.

Adjuvant RT for Patients with pT2 Tumors and Positive Margins

The meaning of positive margins after radical prostatectomy for pT2 carcinomas is controversial. While some authors see no independent prognostic factor for biochemical freedom from disease (bNED), in other studies the positive apical margin with pT2 carcinomas was identified as independent prognostic factor [5, 11]. No randomized studies comparing 'wait and see' and adjuvant RT exist. In only 1 retrospective study on matched pair conditions, 2 cohorts with 76 patients each were compared. The 5-year bNED rate amounted to 88% for the patients with adjuvant RT compared to 59% with wait and see (p < 0.05). No difference between positive basal or apical margins resulted [15]. A randomized comparison is being prepared at present by the Interdisziplinäre Studiengruppe Prostatakarzinom in Germany. In the subgroup analysis of the EORTC 22911 trial, patients

Table 1. Comparison of radical prostatectomy with and without adjuvant RT for pT3 prostate carcinoma – clinical local control

Reference	With RT		Without RT	
	n	5-year local control rate, %	n	5-year local control rate, %
Anscher et al. [17]	46	96	113	80
Wiegel and Bressel [19]	56	100	–	–
Schild et al. [20]	60	100	228	83
Syndikus et al. [21]	89	100	88	79
Petrovich et al. [18]	201	95	–	–

with pT2 R1 tumors were at similar risk of failure as men presenting with extra-capsular extension with or without positive surgical margins but without invasion of seminal vesicles [16]. The indication for adjuvant RT for patients with pT2 prostate cancer and positive margins can be seen to be due to individual risk factors.

Adjuvant RT for pT3 pN0 Tumors with or without Positive Margins

A large number of retrospective, nonrandomized studies is available on this question. In particular, different prognostic factors like positive margins, infiltration of the periprostatic tissue or seminal vesicles and Gleason score >7 were examined. In these retrospective studies with adjuvant RT, a significant improvement in the local tumor control rate, up to 95–100%, was achieved [9, 12, 17–19] (table 1). A number of retrospective researchers also conclude that in the adjuvant situation an RT with 60 Gy results in a significant increase in bNED (table 2). The order of magnitude of this extension on 4–5 years varies between 20 and 50% [12]. In a study by Valicenti et al. [25], a matched pair analysis of 72 patients was performed. In this analysis, patients were grouped according to Gleason score (<7 vs. ≥7), preoperative PSA value (≤10 vs. >10 ng/ml), seminal vesicle infiltration (positive vs. negative) and margin status (positive vs. negative). Five-year freedom from PSA relapse was 89 versus 55% (p < 0.05) in favor of the treated patients. Different authors identified different factors of risk. Clear indications resulted on the fact that sole seminal vesicle infiltration, in particular with negative margins, is not sufficiently treated with adjuvant RT alone [26]. In the majority of cases, positive margins, expanded organ-exceeding tumor growth and a preoperative PSA value >10 ng/ml could be identified [12, 13]. There are inconsistent data on the importance of adjuvant RT for patients with Gleason score 8–10.

Table 2. Comparison of radical prostatectomy with and without adjuvant RT for pT3 prostate carcinoma and 5-year bNED survival – retrospective studies

Reference	With RT		Without RT	
	n	5-year unde-tectable, %	n	5-year unde-tectable, %
Zietman et al. [22]	84	73	62	27
Schild et al. [20]	60	57	228	40
Syndikus et al. [21]	89	93	88	74
Valicenti et al. [25]	36	89	36	55
Choo et al. [23]	73	88	52	65
Vargas et al. [24]	23	52	72	30

In no series, however, could an extension of overall survival be proven. This is probably connected with the number of investigated patients. In order to be able to prove a survival advantage of 5–10%, between 500 and 1,000 patients and a median follow-up of 8–10 years are required. This fact is in particular verified from the RTOG studies [27].

Randomized Trials

To date, data from 3 randomized phase III studies have been presented, including the EORTC 22911 study and a study by the Southwest Oncology Group (SWOG) [16, 17, 28]. Another study is available only in abstract form at present [13]. In principle, all 3 studies are positive. They uniformly show an absolute advantage in bNED of about 20% after 4–5 years.

In the EORTC study, 1,002 patients were randomized to RT with 60 Gy or 'wait and see', and the results were published by Bolla et al. [29]. The median PSA value before the beginning of RT was 0.2 ng/ml, indicating an unfavorable patient selection. After 5 years, bNED for irradiated patients was 74% compared with 52.6% in the control arm (p < 0.05) [16, 29]. The absolute advantage by RT was 21%. In parallel to this, the rate of locoregional recurrences, diagnosed by clinical palpation, was significantly reduced by adjuvant RT. The relevance of this is limited, however, because of the merely clinical palpation, which gives a false positive in up to 30% [29].

The study of the Arbeitsgemeinschaften Radiologische Onkologie und Urologische Onkologie der Deutschen Krebsgesellschaft (ARO 96-02/AUO AP 09/95) differ in that the condition for entrance and randomization into 'wait and see' or adjuvant RT with 60 Gy was undetecable PSA after radical prostatectomy. Three hundred and eighty five patients were randomized, 78 of these did not reach the undetectable PSA range and were excluded according to the study protocol. The remaining 307 patients were randomized into 'wait and see' (n = 153) and adjuvant RT with 60 Gy (n = 154). The median follow-up was 40 months. After 4 years, a significant advantage of 21% for bNED was observed [13].

In the randomized phase III study by SWOG, which was started in the pre-PSA era, the primary endpoint was an expected advantage for metastasis-free survival after 10 years. This primary endpoint was not reached, the study thus regarding the primary endpoint negatively. After 10 years, however, there was a significant advantage for bNED for adjuvant RT (38 vs. 23%; absolute difference 15%) [16].

While a significant advantage for bNED was proven in all 3 studies, there is at present no advantage in overall survival. A randomized study with patients only irradiated for rising PSA after radical prostatectomy does not exist. It is for these reasons justifiable to treat patients with positive margins after radical prostatectomy with adjuvant RT with 60 Gy.

Acute and Late Side Effects of Adjuvant RT

The rate of severe acute and late side effects after adjuvant RT with 60 Gy is low. In the German multicenter study, the rate of severe grade III acute or late side effects was below 1%, because all irradiated patients had undergone three-dimensional treatment planning [13]. Low grade I/II side effects involving the rectum and bladder occur in up to 5–15% of patients, but doses at about 60 Gy given in the frame of three-dimensional RT treatment planning are rarely associated with serious long-term side effects (less than 3–4% grade III/IV according to the RTOG-EORTC grading system) [12, 16, 17, 29]. It is important that adjuvant RT does not have a negative influence on continence after radical prostatectomy. To date, no data exist on the question of a loss of sexual potency after nerve-sparing radical prostatectomy and adjuvant RT. This problem will more frequently arise in the future with patients with pT2 R1 resections, who today often receive nerve-sparing radical prostatectomy.

In summary, there is a well-documented indication for adjuvant RT for pT3 carcinomas with positive margins, both after reaching an undetectable PSA with persisting PSA after radical prostatectomy, whereby the total dose should then be at least 66 Gy. The indication for adjuvant RT for patients with pT2 prostate cancer and positive margins can be seen due to individual criteria, even if no randomized data exist at present. On the other hand, there is no survival advantage for irradiated patients. It still remains to be examined whether adjuvant RT is superior to RT for rising PSA. The rate of severe late side effects is low.

References

1 Chun FK, Graefen M, Zacharias M, Haese A, Steuber T, Schlomm T, Walz J, Karakiewicz PI, Huland H: Anatomic radical retropubic prostatectomy – long-term recurrence-free survival rates for localized prostate cancer. World J Urol 2006;24:273–280.

2 Partin AW, Mangold LA, Lamm DM, Walsh PC, Epstein JI, Pearson JD: Contemporary update of prostate cancer staging nomograms (Partin Tables) for the new millennium. Urology 2001;58:843–848.

3 Roehl KA, Han M, Ramos CG, Antenor JA, Catalona WJ: Cancer progression and survival rates following anatomical radical retropubic prostatectomy in 3,478 consecutive patients: long-term results. J Urol 2004;172:910–914.

4 Morgan WR, Bergstralh EJ, Zincke H: Long-term evaluation of radical prostatectomy as treatment for clinical stage C (T3) prostate cancer. Urology 1993;41:116–120.

5 Pinto F, Prayer-Galetti T, Gardiman M, Sacco E, Ciaccia M, Fracalanza S, Betto G, Pagano F: Clinical and pathological characteristics of patients presenting with biochemical progression after radical retropubic prostatectomy for pathologically organ-confined prostate cancer. Urol Int 2006;76:202–208.

6 Stephenson AJ, Scardino PT, Eastham JA, Bianco FJ Jr, Dotan ZA, Fearn PA, Kattan MW: Preoperative nomogram predicting the 10-year probability of prostate cancer recurrence after radical prostatectomy. J Natl Cancer Inst 2006;17:715–717.

7 Swindle P, Eastham JA, Ohori M, Kattan MW, Wheeler T, Maru N, Slawin K, Scardino PT: Do margins matter? The prognostic significance of positive surgical margins in radical prostatectomy specimens. J Urol 2005;174:903–907.

8 Shekarriz B, Upadhyay J, Wood DP Jr, Hinman J, Raasch J, Cummings GD, Grignon D, Littrup PJ: Vesicourethral anastomosis biopsy after radical prostatectomy: predictive value of prostate-specific antigen and pathologic stage. Urology 1999;54:1044–1048.

9 Morris MM, Dallow KC, Zietman AL: Adjuvant and salvage irradiation following radical prostatectomy for prostate cancer. Int J Radiat Oncol Biol Phys 1997;38:731–736.

10 Pazona JF, Han M, Hawkins SA, Roehl KA, Catalona WJ: Salvage radiation therapy for prostate specific antigen progression following radical prostatectomy: 10-year outcome estimates. J Urol 2005;174:1282–1286.

11 Salomon L, Anastasiadis AG, Antiphon P, Levrel O, Saint F, De La Taille A, Cicco A, Vordos D, Hoznek A, Chopin D, Abbou CC: Prognostic consequences of the location of positive surgical margins in organ-confined prostate cancer. Urol Int 2003;70:291–296.

12 Teh BS, Bastasch MD, Mai WY, Kattan MW, Butler EB, Kadmon D: Long-term benefits of elective radiotherapy after prostatectomy for patients with positive surgical margins. J Urol 2006;175:2097–2101.

13 Wiegel T, Bottke D, Willich N, Piechota H, Souchon R, Stoeckle M, Ruebe C, Hinke A, Hinkelbein W, Miller K: Phase III results of adjuvant radiotherapy (RT) versus 'wait and see' (WS) in patients with pT3 prostate cancer following radical prostatectomy (RP) (ARO 96–02/AUO AP 09/95). J Clin Oncol 2005;23(suppl):4513.

14 Pollack A, Zagars GK, Starkschall G: Prostate cancer radiation dose response: results of the M.D. Anderson phase III randomized trial. Int J Radiat Oncol Biol Phys 2002;53:1097–1105.

15 Leibovich BC, Engen DE, Patterson DE, Pisansky TM, Alexander EE, Blute ML, Bergstralh EJ, Zincke H: Benefit of adjuvant radiation therapy for localized prostate cancer with a positive surgical margin. J Urol 2000;163:1189–1190.

16 Collette L, van Poppel H, Bolla M, van Cangh P, Vekemans K, Da Pozzo L, de Reijke TM, Verbaeys A, Bosset JF, Pierart M, European Organisation for Research and Treatment of Cancer (EORTC) Radiotherapy and Genito-urinary Groups: Patients at high risk of progression after radical prostatectomy: do they all benefit from immediate post-operative irradiation? (EORTC trial 22911). Eur J Cancer 2005;41:2662–2672.

17 Anscher MS, Robertson CN, Prosnitz LR: Adjuvant radiotherapy for pathologic stage T3/4 adenocarcinoma of the prostate: ten-year update. Int J Radiat Oncol Biol Phys 1995;33:37–43.

18 Petrovich Z, Lieskovsky G, Langholz B: Radical prostatectomy and post-operative irradiation in patients with pathological stage C (T3) carcinoma of the prostate. Int J Radiat Oncol Biol Phys 1998;40:139–147.

19 Wiegel T, Bressel M: Adjuvant radiotherapy following radical prostatectomy – results of 56 patients. Eur J Cancer 1995;31A:5–11.

20 Schild SE, Wong WW, Grado GL: The results of radical retropubic prostatectomy and adjuvant therapy for pathological stage C prostate cancer. Int J Radiat Oncol Biol Phys 1996;34:535–541.

21 Syndikus I, Pickles T, Kostashuk E: Postoperative radiotherapy for stage pT3 carcinoma of the prostate: improved local control. J Urol 1996;155: 1983–1986.

22 Zietman AL, Coen JJ, Shipley WU, Althausen AF: Adjuvant irradiation after radical prostatectomy for adenocarcinoma of prostate: analysis of freedom from PSA failure. Urology 1993;42:292–298.

23 Choo R, Hruby G, Hong J, Hong E, DeBoer G, Danjoux C, Morton G, Klotz L, Bhak E, Flavin A: Positive resection margin and/or pathologic T3 adenocarcinoma of prostate with undetectable postoperative prostate-specific antigen after radical prostatectomy: to irradiate or not? Int J Radiat Oncol Biol Phys 2002;52:674–680.

24 Vargas C, Kestin LL, Weed DW, Krauss D, Vicini FA, Martinez AA: Improved biochemical outcome with adjuvant radiotherapy after radical prostatectomy for prostate cancer with poor pathologic features. Int J Radiat Oncol Biol Phys 2005;61:714–724.

25 Valicenti RK, Gomella LG, Ismail M: The efficacy of early adjuvant radiation therapy for pT3N0 prostate cancer: a matched pair analysis. Int J Radiat Oncol Biol Phys 1999;45:53–58.

26 Eggener SE, Roehl KA, Smith ND, Antenor JA, Han M, Catalona WJ: Contemporary survival results and the role of radiation therapy in patients with node negative seminal vesicle invasion following radical prostatectomy. J Urol 2005;173: 1150–1155.

27 Pilepich MV, Winter K, Lawton CA, Krisch RE, Wolkov HB, Movsas B, Hug EB, Asbell SO, Grignon D: Androgen suppression adjuvant to definitive radiotherapy in prostate carcinoma – long-term results of phase III RTOG 85-31. Int J Radiat Oncol Biol Phys 2005;61:1285–1290.

28 Thompson IM Jr, Tangen CM, Paradelo J, Lucia MS, Miller G, Troyer D, Messing E, Forman J, Chin J, Swanson G, Canby-Hagino E, Crawford ED: Adjuvant radiotherapy for pathologically advanced prostate cancer: results of a clinical trial. JAMA 2006;296:2329–2335.

29 Bolla M, van Poppel H, Collette L, van Cangh P, Vekemans K, Da Pozzo L, de Reijke TM, Verbaeys A, Bosset JF, van Velthoven R, Marechal JM, Scalliet P, Haustermans K, Pierart M, European Organization for Research and Treatment of Cancer: Postoperative radiotherapy after radical prostatectomy: a randomised controlled trial (EORTC trial 22911). Lancet 2005;366:572–578.

Prof. Thomas Wiegel
Department of Radiotherapy and Radiation Oncology, University Hospital Ulm
Robert-Koch-Strasse 6
DE–89081 Ulm (Germany)
Tel. +49 731 500 56101, Fax +49 731 500 56110, E-Mail thomas.wiegel@uniklinik-ulm.de

Moser L, Schostak M, Miller K, Hinkelbein W (eds): Controversies in the Treatment of
Prostate Cancer. Front Radiat Ther Oncol. Basel, Karger, 2008, vol 41, pp 39–48

Adjuvant Hormonal Treatment – The Bicalutamide Early Prostate Cancer Program

Manfred P. Wirth   Oliver W. Hakenberg   Michael Froehner

Department of Urology, University Hospital Carl Gustav Carus, Technical University of Dresden,
Dresden, Germany

Abstract

Several randomized trials have demonstrated that adjuvant medical or surgical castration may improve overall survival in patients with locally advanced prostate cancer undergoing external beam
radiotherapy. After radical prostatectomy, patients with positive lymph nodes seem to benefit from
adjuvant hormonal treatment rather than from treatment at the time of clinical progression in terms
of overall survival. In patients with locally advanced, lymph node-negative prostate cancer, adjuvant
hormonal treatment after radical prostatectomy has been demonstrated to delay progression without impact on survival. The Bicalutamide Early Prostate Cancer Program, the largest ongoing prostate cancer trial in the world, investigates the effect of early treatment with 150 mg bicalutamide
compared with placebo as monotherapy or adjuvant treatment after radical prostatectomy or external beam radiotherapy. It demonstrated that early treatment with bicalutamide may delay objective progression of prostate cancer irrespective of primary treatment. Considering overall survival, however, there was an advantage only in the setting of external beam radiotherapy for
locally advanced prostate cancer. In patients with localized disease who initially underwent watchful waiting, there was a trend to decreased survival in the arm immediately treated with bicalutamide. Altogether, there is no indication for treatment with bicalutamide in patients with localized
disease.

Prostate cancer is currently the second most commonly diagnosed nondermato-
logical malignancy in men and the most common one in developed countries [1].
It has been estimated that about half of the patients experience prostate-specific
antigen (PSA) failure within 10 years after receiving any type of local treatment

Prof. M.P. Wirth is the principal investigator of the 'Bicalutamide Early Prostate Cancer Program', which is
supported by AstraZeneca.

for prostate cancer [2]. Efforts have been undertaken to investigate the effect of early (adjuvant and neoadjuvant) hormonal manipulations [3]. Nevertheless, optimal dose, time and duration of hormonal therapy adjuvant to curative treatment are still unknown [4]. This article summarizes the current knowledge on adjuvant treatment of prostate cancer with a special focus on radiotherapy and the Bicalutamide Early Prostate Cancer Program.

Adjuvant Hormonal Treatment after Radical Prostatectomy

At present, definite evidence from randomized studies supporting immediate (adjuvant) endocrine treatment after radical prostatectomy is still pending. Retrospective studies found a survival advantage for adjuvant hormonal treatment in patients with positive lymph nodes and diploid disease and in patients with seminal vesical involvement [5, 6]. However, in one, relatively small randomized trial (n = 98), adjuvant hormonal treatment was compared with observation until clinical progression in patients with minimal lymph node disease after pelvic lymph node dissection and radical prostatectomy. Disease-specific and overall mortality were significantly better in patients treated with adjuvant androgen deprivation [7, 8]. Other studies revealed, however, conflicting results. A larger study (n = 302) in patients with stage D1 disease who did not undergo radical prostatectomy showed no advantage for immediate hormonal treatment, compared with deferred treatment [9]. Furthermore, retrospective studies in radical prostatectomy patients with positive lymph nodes found much less clear differences [5]. We performed a multicenter randomized trial with locally advanced, lymph node-negative prostate cancer (n = 352). Group 1 received adjuvant treatment with flutamide, whereas group 2 received no immediate treatment. The decision to start or to change treatment at relapse or adverse events rested with the patients and their physicians. Tumor progression was delayed in the flutamide arm (p = 0.0041). There was, however, no difference in overall survival after a median follow-up of 6.1 years (p = 0.92) [10].

Adjuvant Hormonal Treatment after Radiotherapy

A great amount of data from randomized trials supports adjuvant hormonal treatment after external beam radiotherapy for locally advanced prostate cancer (table 1). It has been demonstrated that adjuvant hormonal therapy started with radiotherapy significantly improves disease-specific and overall survival in this setting (table 2). Overall, high-risk patients seem to benefit from immediate androgen deprivation after external beam radiotherapy, whereas in earlier stages the differ-

Table 1. Effect of adjuvant hormonal treatment after radiotherapy: overview of prospective randomized trials

Authors	Stages	Regimen	Progression	Survival
Bolla et al. [11, 12]	T1–T4N0–x	LHRH analogs	advantage for adjuvant treatment	advantage for adjuvant treatment
Pilepich et al. [13, 14], Lawton et al. [15]	stage C or D1	LHRH analogs	advantage for adjuvant treatment	advantage for adjuvant treatment
Granfors et al. [16]	T1–4N0–1	orchiectomy	advantage for adjuvant treatment	advantage for adjuvant treatment in N1 subgroup
Hanks et al. [17]	T2b–T4, PSA <150 ng/ml	LHRH analogs plus flutamide	advantage for adjuvant treatment	advantage for adjuvant treatment in Gleason score 8–10 subgroup
D'Amico et al. [18]	Gleason score 7+, cT3–4 or PSA ≥10 ng/ml	LHRH analogs	advantage for adjuvant treatment	advantage for adjuvant treatment
Wirth et al. [20], McLeod et al. [21]	T1b–T4 N0–1M0	bicalutamide	advantage for adjuvant treatment	advantage for adjuvant treatment only in locally advanced disease

Survival advantage has mainly been observed in patients with advanced disease and a high risk of early distant progression. LHRH = Luteinizing hormone-releasing hormone.

ences tend to diminish [23]. It is, however, still unknown, whether the observed survival advantages could also be obtained by hormonal therapy alone, since such a control arm was not included in these studies.

Antiandrogen Monotherapy for Nonmetastatic Locally Advanced and Metastatic Prostate Cancer

Nonsteroidal antiandrogens (bicalutamide, flutamide, nilutamide) competitively inhibit the activity of androgens at the androgen receptor and maintain or even increase the serum testosterone level. Bicalutamide is considered to be the best-tolerated and most extensively studied drug in this group [24–26]. Compared with

Table 2. Effect of adjuvant hormonal treatment after radical prostatectomy: overview of prospective randomized trials

Authors	Stages	Regimen	Progression	Survival
Messing et al. [7, 8]	pN+	orchiectomy or LHRH analogs	advantage for adjuvant treatment	advantage for adjuvant treatment
Prayer-Galetti et al. [19]	stage C	LHRH analogs	advantage for adjuvant treatment	not available
Wirth et al. [10]	pT3–4pN0	flutamide	advantage for adjuvant treatment	no difference
Wirth et al. [20, 22], McLeod et al. [21]	T1b–T4 N0–1M0	bicalutamide	advantage for adjuvant treatment	no difference

Only 1 study has demonstrated a survival advantage for adjuvant treatment to date.
LHRH = Luteinizing hormone-releasing hormone.

medical castration, bicalutamide monotherapy has been found to increase bone density, to lessen fat accumulation and to have fewer bothersome adverse effects [27, 28]. Gynecomastia and breast pain are frequent side effects of bicalutamide monotherapy [24, 29].

In 2 combined randomized trials involving 480 patients with locally advanced nonmetastatic disease (clinical stages T3–T4M0), bicalutamide monotherapy (150 mg daily) was compared with castration. After a median follow-up of 6.3 years, there was no detectable difference between bicalutamide monotherapy and castration concerning time to progression and overall survival. Advantages for bicalutamide monotherapy were observed concerning sexual interest and physical capacity. Detailed data on sexual potency have, however, not been reported. Other data suggest that approximately one third of patients receiving 150 mg bicalutamide daily maintain sexual function during treatment [30].

Tyrrell et al. [31] compared bicalutamide monotherapy (150 mg daily) with castration as treatment for locally advanced nonmetastatic or metastatic prostate cancer (n = 1,453). Bicalutamide monotherapy was as effective as castration in nonmetastatic patients, but there was a small survival advantage for castration in the M1 subgroup. This difference was partially outweighed by a better tolerability profile and a higher quality of life in patients treated with bicalutamide mono-

therapy [31]. Altogether, bicalutamide monotherapy is an option for patients with locally advanced prostate cancer as well as in selected patients with metastatic disease. In men with a high tumor burden (that is, PSA values greater than 400 ng/ml), it is, however, inferior to castration [32].

The Bicalutamide Early Prostate Cancer Program

The Bicalutamide Early Prostate Cancer Program is the largest ongoing prostate cancer trial in the world, comprising 8,113 patients. In this program, the nonsteroidal antiandrogen bicalutamide is being evaluated as primary or adjuvant treatment for early prostate cancer [comprising the clinical tumor stages T1b–4N0–1M0, subdivided into localized (T1–2, N0/Nx) or locally advanced (T3–4, any N; any T, N+) prostate cancer]. The program consists of 3 double-blind, parallel-group trials [1 in North America (trial 23, n = 3,292), 1 in Mexico, South Africa, Australia and Europe (trial 24, n = 3,603) and 1 in Scandinavia (trial 25, n = 1,218)] [22]. In the North American trial, all patients underwent curative treatment (radical prostatectomy or radiotherapy) prior to study entry. In trials 24 and 25, expectant management was allowed as primary treatment beside radical prostatectomy and radiotherapy [20, 22]. The patients were randomized to receive either placebo (n = 4,061) or bicalutamide 150 mg once daily (n = 4,052). In the North American trial, more than 70% of patients had a disease stage of less than T3, compared with about 60% in the European and Scandinavian trials. In the North American trial, more than 80% of patients had undergone radical prostatectomy and only 20% received radiotherapy prior to randomization, compared to 46 and 18%, respectively, in the Mexico, South Africa, Australia and Europe trial. In the Scandinavian trial, only 13% of patients enrolled underwent radical prostatectomy and only 5% underwent radiotherapy. The study treatment was given for 2 years in the American trial and until disease progression in the other 2 trials of the program. A maximum treatment duration of 5 years was recommended in the European trial [29, 21]. Time to objective clinical progression (defined as tumor progression confirmed by either biopsy, ultrasound, computerized tomography, bone scan or magnetic resonance imaging, or death of any cause) and survival were the primary study endpoints. Time to treatment failure (discontinuation of treatment), PSA progression (defined as doubling of the PSA value measured immediately prior to the first application of the study medication) and toxicity were defined as secondary study endpoints. After a median follow-up of 7.4 years, 29.3% of patients in the bicalutamide arm and 10.0% in the placebo arm withdrew from the randomized treatment because of adverse effects, whereas disease progression was the reason for withdrawal in 5.5% of patients in the bicalutamide arm and in 12.9% in the placebo arm [21]. Breast pain (73.6%) and gynecomastia

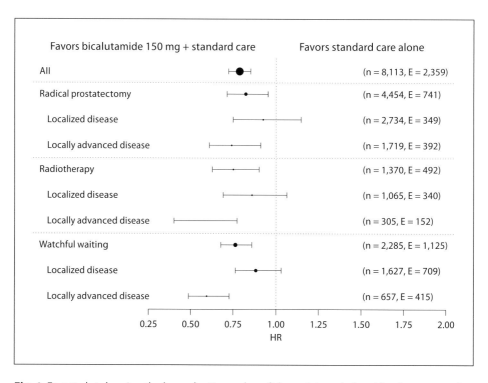

Fig. 1. Forest plot showing the hazard ratios and confidence intervals for objective progression in the Bicalutamide Early Prostate Cancer Program stratified by primary treatment and disease stage. E = Total number of events; n = number of patients in each subgroup; HR = hazard ratio [21]. Reprinted with permission from Blackwell Publishing.

(68.8%) were the most frequent side effects in the bicalutamide arm. These side effects were mild or moderate in more than 90% of cases. At the time of the most recently published analysis, at a median follow-up of 7.4 years, there was no benefit concerning progression-free survival by adding bicalutamide to standard care in localized disease (fig. 1) [21]. There was even a trend towards decreased overall survival in patients with localized prostate cancer undergoing watchful waiting when treated with bicalutamide (hazard ratio 1.16, 95% confidence interval 0.99–1.37, p = 0.07; fig. 2). In those with locally advanced disease, however, bicalutamide significantly improved progression-free survival irrespective of primary treatment applied (fig. 1). In patients initially treated by radiotherapy, bicalutamide significantly improved overall survival (hazard ratio 0.65, 95% confidence interval 0.44–0.95, p = 0.03, fig. 2–4) due to a lower risk of prostate cancer-related mortality. There was a trend towards improved overall survival in patients with locally advanced disease undergoing watchful waiting receiving bicalutamide (hazard ratio 0.81, 95% confidence interval 0.66–1.01, p = 0.06, fig. 2). No surviv-

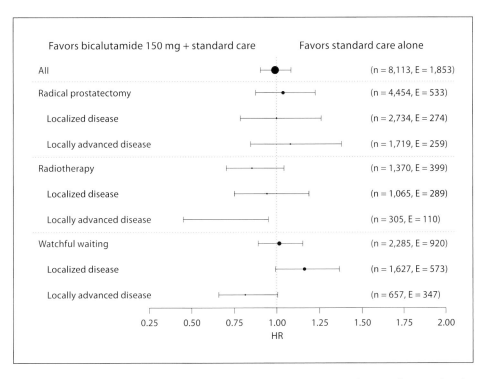

Fig. 2. Forest plot showing the hazard ratios and confidence intervals for overall survival in the Bicalutamide Early Prostate Cancer Program stratified by primary treatment and disease stage. E = Total number of events; n = number of patients in each subgroup; HR = hazard ratio [21]. Reprinted with permission from Blackwell Publishing.

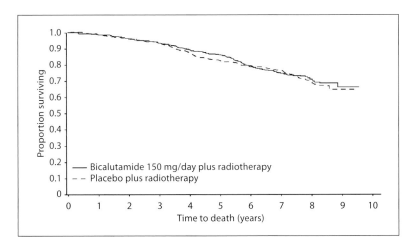

Fig. 3. Overall survival after radiotherapy for localized prostate cancer (n = 1,065). There was no difference between patients with or without bicalutamide treatment (hazard ratio 0.94, 95% confidence interval 0.75–1.19, p = 0.63) [33]. Reprinted with permission from Springer Verlag.

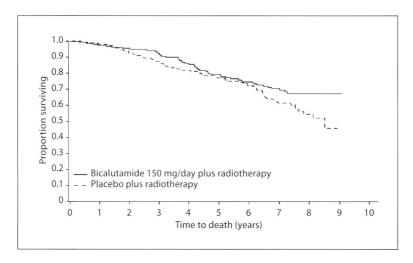

Fig. 4. Overall survival after radiotherapy for locally advanced prostate cancer (n = 305). There was a significant advantage for adjuvant treatment with bicalutamide (hazard ratio 0.65, 95% confidence interval 0.44–0.95, p = 0.03) [33]. Reprinted with permission from Springer Verlag.

al difference was seen in the radical prostatectomy subgroup (fig. 2). Overall, the currently available data from the Bicalutamide Early Prostate Cancer Program suggest that early or adjuvant hormonal therapy is not appropriate for patients with localized disease [21, 26].

Conclusion

The Bicalutamide Early Prostate Cancer Program demonstrated that early treatment with bicalutamide may delay objective progression of prostate cancer irrespective of the way the tumor had initially been treated. Considering overall survival, however, there was an advantage only in the setting of external beam radiotherapy for locally advanced prostate cancer. In patients with localized disease who initially underwent watchful waiting, there was a trend to decreased survival in the arm immediately treated with bicalutamide. Altogether, patients with localized disease did not benefit from early treatment with bicalutamide.

References

1 Parkin DM, Bray F, Ferlay J, Pisani P: Global cancer statistics, 2002. CA Cancer J Clin 2005;55: 74–108.

2 Walsh PC, DeWeese TL, Eisenberger MA: A structured debate: immediate versus deferred androgen suppression in prostate cancer – evidence for deferred treatment. J Urol 2001;166:508–515.

3 Ryan CJ, Small EJ: Early versus delayed androgen deprivation for prostate cancer: new fuel for an old debate. J Clin Oncol 2005;23:8225–8231.

4 Jani AB, Hellman S: Early prostate cancer: clinical decision-making. Lancet 2003;361:1045–1053.

5 Seay TM, Blute ML, Zincke H: Long-term outcome in patients with pTxN+ adenocarcinoma of prostate treated with radical prostatectomy and early androgen ablation. J Urol 1998;159:357–364.

6 Zincke H, Lau W, Bergstralh E, Blute ML: Role of early adjuvant hormonal therapy after radical prostatectomy for prostate cancer. J Urol 2001; 166:2208–2215.

7 Messing EM, Manola J, Sarosdy M, Wilding G, Crawford ED, Trump D: Immediate hormonal therapy compared with observation after radical prostatectomy and pelvic lymphadenectomy in men with node-positive prostate cancer. N Engl J Med 1999;341:1781–1788.

8 Messing EM, Manola J, Yao J, Kiernan M, Crawford D, Wilding G, et al: Immediate versus deferred androgen deprivation treatment in patients with node-positive prostate cancer after radical prostatectomy and pelvic lymphadenectomy. Lancet Oncol 2006;7:472–479.

9 Schroder FH, Kurth KH, Fossa SD, Hoekstra W, Karthaus PP, Debois M, et al: Early versus delayed endocrine treatment of pN1–3 M0 prostate cancer without local treatment of the primary tumor: results of European Organisation for the Research and Treatment of Cancer 30846 – a phase III study. J Urol 2004;172:923–927.

10 Wirth MP, Weissbach L, Marx FJ, Heckl W, Jellinghaus W, Riedmiller H, et al: Prospective randomized trial comparing flutamide as adjuvant treatment versus observation after radical prostatectomy for locally advanced, lymph node-negative prostate cancer. Eur Urol 2004;45:267–270.

11 Bolla M, Gonzalez D, Warde P, Dubois JB, Mirimanoff RO, Storme G, et al: Improved survival in patients with locally advanced prostate cancer treated with radiotherapy and goserelin. N Engl J Med 1997;337:295–300.

12 Bolla M, Collette L, Blank L, Warde P, Dubois JB, Mirimanoff RO, et al: Long-term results with immediate androgen suppression and external irradiation in patients with locally advanced prostate cancer (an EORTC study): a phase III randomised trial. Lancet 2002;360:103–106.

13 Pilepich MV, Caplan R, Byhardt RW, Lawton CA, Gallagher MJ, Mesic JB, et al: Phase III trial of androgen suppression using goserelin in unfavorable-prognosis carcinoma of the prostate treated with definitive radiotherapy: report of Radiation Therapy Oncology Group Protocol 85-31. J Clin Oncol 1997;15:1013–1021.

14 Pilepich MV, Winter K, John MJ, Mesic JB, Sause W, Rubin P, et al: Phase III radiation therapy oncology group (RTOG) trial 86-10 of androgen deprivation adjuvant to definitive radiotherapy in locally advanced carcinoma of the prostate. Int J Radiat Oncol Biol Phys 2001;50:1243–1252.

15 Lawton CA, Winter K, Murray K, Machtay M, Mesic JB, Hanks GE, et al: Updated results of the phase III Radiation Therapy Oncology Group (RTOG) trial 85-31 evaluating the potential benefit of androgen suppression following standard radiation therapy for unfavorable prognosis carcinoma of the prostate. Int J Radiat Oncol Biol Phys 2001;49:937–946.

16 Granfors T, Modig H, Damber JE, Tomic R: Long-term follow-up of a randomized study of locally advanced prostate cancer treated with combined orchiectomy and external radiotherapy versus radiotherapy alone. J Urol 2006;176: 544–547.

17 Hanks GE, Pajak TF, Porter A, Grignon D, Brereton H, Venkatesan V, et al: Phase III trial of long-term adjuvant androgen deprivation after neoadjuvant hormonal cytoreduction and radiotherapy in locally advanced carcinoma of the prostate: the Radiation Therapy Oncology Group Protocol 92-02. J Clin Oncol 2003;21:3972–3978.

18 D'Amico AV, Manola J, Loffredo M, Renshaw AA, DellaCroce A, Kantoff PW. 6-month androgen suppression plus radiation therapy vs radiation therapy alone for patients with clinically localized prostate cancer: a randomized controlled trial. JAMA 2004;292:821–827.

19 Prayer-Galetti T, Zattoni F, Capizzi A, Dal Moro F, Pagano F, et al: Disease-free survival in patients with pathological 'C stage' prostate cancer at radical retropubic prostatectomy submitted to adjuvant hormonal treatment. Eur Urol 2000; 38(suppl 4):504.

20 Wirth M, Tyrrell C, Wallace M, Delaere KP, Sanchez-Chapado M, Ramon J, et al: Bicalutamide (Casodex) 150 mg as immediate therapy in patients with localized or locally advanced prostate cancer significantly reduces the risk of disease progression. Urology 2001;58:146–151.

21 McLeod DG, Iversen P, See WA, Morris T, Armstrong J, Wirth MP, et al: Bicalutamide 150 mg plus standard care vs standard care alone for early prostate cancer. BJU Int 2006;97:247–254.

22 Wirth M, Tyrrell C, Delaere K, Sanchez-Chapado M, Ramon J WD, Hetherington J, et al: Bicalutamide ('Casodex') 150 mg in addition to standard care in patients with nonmetastatic prostate cancer: updated results from a randomised double-blind phase III study (median follow-up 5.1 y) in the early prostate cancer programme. Prostate Cancer Prostatic Dis 2005;8:194–200.

23 Sharifi N, Gulley JL, Dahut WL: Androgen deprivation therapy for prostate cancer. JAMA 2005; 294:238–244.

24 Iversen P: Bicalutamide monotherapy for early state prostate cancer. J Urol 2003;170:S48–S54.

25 Aus G, Abbou CC, Heidenreich A, Schmid HP, van Poppel H, Wolff J, et al: EAU guidelines on prostate cancer. Eur Urol 2005;48:546–551.

26 Wirth MP, Hakenberg OW, Froehner M: Antiandrogens in the treatment of prostate cancer. Eur Urol 2007;51:306–313.

27 Smith MR, Goode M, Zietman AL, McGovern FJ, Lee H, Finkelstein JS: Bicalutamide monotherapy versus leuprolide monotherapy for prostate cancer: effects on bone mineral density and body composition. J Clin Oncol 2004;22:2546–2553.

28 Sieber PR, Keiller DL, Kahnoski RJ, Gallo J, McFadden S: Bicalutamide 150 mg maintains bone mineral density during monotherapy for localized or locally advanced prostate cancer. J Urol 2004;171:2272–2276.

29 Wirth MP, See WA, McLeod DG, Iversen P, Morris T, Carroll K, et al: Bicalutamide 150 mg in addition to standard care in patients with localized or locally advanced prostate cancer: results from the second analysis of the early prostate cancer program at median follow-up of 5.4 years. J Urol 2004;172:1865–1870.

30 Iversen P, Tyrrell CJ, Kaisary AV, Anderson JB, van Poppel H, Tammela TLJ, et al: Bicalutamide monotherapy compared with castration in patients with nonmetastatic locally advanced prostate cancer: 6.3 years of followup. J Urol 2000; 164:1579–1582.

31 Tyrrell CJ, Kaisary AV, Iversen P, Anderson JB, Baert L, Tammela T, et al. A randomised comparison of 'Casodex' (bicalutamide) 150 mg monotherapy versus castration in the treatment of metastatic and locally advanced prostate cancer. Eur Urol 1998;33:447–456.

32 Kolvenbag GJ, Iversen P, Newling DW: Antiandrogen monotherapy: a new form of treatment for patients with prostate cancer. Urology 2001; 58:16–23.

33 See WA, Tyrrell CJ, CASODEX Early Prostate Cancer Trialists' Group: The addition of bicalutamide 150 mg to radiotherapy significantly improves overall survival in men with locally advanced prostate cancer. J Cancer Res Clin Oncol 2006;132(suppl 13):S7–S16.

Prof. Manfred P. Wirth
Department of Urology
University Hospital Carl Gustav Carus, Technical University of Dresden
Fetscherstrasse 74
DE–01307 Dresden (Germany)
Tel. +49 351 458 2447, Fax +49 351 458 4333, E-Mail Manfred.Wirth@uniklinikum-dresden.de

Moser L, Schostak M, Miller K, Hinkelbein W (eds): Controversies in the Treatment of
Prostate Cancer. Front Radiat Ther Oncol. Basel, Karger, 2008, vol 41, pp 49–57

Hormone Therapy for Prostate Cancer – Immediate Initiation

M. Schostak   K. Miller   M. Schrader

Department of Urology, Charité Universitätsmedizin Berlin, Berlin, Germany

Abstract

Although hormone therapy is widely used in the management of prostate cancer, the optimal timing of its initiation remains a matter of debate. Many studies of the last decades have reported a small
but significant survival benefit and a clear delay in the development of clinical symptoms after early
initiation of therapy. Patients who have localized or locally advanced prostate cancer and are not
suitable for curative options like radical prostatectomy or radiotherapy can best be managed by
hormone therapy alone, which has already been recognized as the optimal treatment for metastatic disease. On the other hand, long-term hormone treatment will expose the patient to the risk of
substantial adverse effects, including muscle wasting, chronic fatigue and osteoporosis. Prognostic
and quality-of-life factors also have an impact on the treatment decision, particularly in patients most
likely to profit from an extension of the remaining life span. Based on available evidence, early hormone therapy may be recommended for men with poorly differentiated tumors or advanced disease
and for those infrequently seen by their physicians. This management can prevent prostate cancer
from migrating to the bones, where treatment becomes extremely difficult and cure or even long-
term control of the disease is an exception.   Copyright © 2008 S. Karger AG, Basel

Charles B. Huggins received the 1966 Nobel Prize in Medicine for his discovery
that hormone withdrawal by orchiectomy or contrasexual treatment can stop the
growth of prostate cancer. This endocrine therapy of prostate cancer has since
been applied when other treatment options like prostatectomy or radiotherapy
cannot be performed or are rejected by the patient. This applies not only to the
localized stage, but also particularly to locally advanced or metastatic prostate
cancer [1, 2].

The disadvantage of orchiectomy is, however, the irreversibility of the surgical measure. The first oral antiandrogens were developed and approved in the late 1960s and early 1970s. The most important one was diethylstilbestrol (DES). Apart from the side effects of hormone withdrawal, DES caused severe cardiovascular toxicity that must be characterized as virtually lethal [3]. This formed the basis for large studies to determine how long the therapy can be deferred before the patient suffers decisive disadvantages from the delay. This controversy has not yet been definitively resolved due to the particularly slow growth of prostate cancer.

The results of 2 large European studies have been published within the last 2 years. They deal with survival differences between patients with immediate and delayed initiation of hormone withdrawal in prostate cancer patients. The patients in these studies were either medically unsuitable for curative therapy or had rejected it [4, 5]. Considering these results and those of older studies, arguments in favor of an immediate initiation of therapy in these cases are discussed below.

Survival

The large studies initiated in the 1960s and 1970s showed that immediate initiation of therapy offered a small but significant survival advantage after 10 years. Naturally, there were great differences in progression-free survival. The American Society of Clinical Oncology recommends immediate therapy based on a meta-analysis of the Cochrane Collaboration, which examines this question in the 4 largest studies, with a total of 2,176 patients [6, 7]. Table 1 shows the results of important studies.

Though small, the significant differences in total survival have a strong psychological impact: the patient ultimately faces the choice of dying 'in any case', for example of heart disease, or sooner of untreated cancer. The mental stress of this alternative currently seems hard to convey, at least in Germany. A study published in 1998 by Tsevat et al. [8] investigated whether hospital patients over the age of 80 were prepared to relinquish part of their future life span if instead they could be in the best of health for the rest of their life. It turned out that 68.6% would not relinquish a single day or would relinquish a month at most. A long life appears to be more important than a high quality of life [8].

Is Curative Therapy no Longer Possible?

Radical prostatectomy is the oldest type of therapy for prostate cancer and the current gold standard for younger patients. This intervention is subject to age-dependent limits. The operation is associated with an increased risk of inconti-

Table 1. Total survival and progression-free interval in various studies

Study	n	Type of hormone therapy	Overall survival
Mayo [38]	707	adjuvant after RPX (pT3B pN0): OX or LHRH	NA
MRC [39]	934	OX or LHRH	30 vs. 22.8% (sign.)
VACURG II (M0) [40]	294	DES 0.2 mg; DES 1 mg; DES 5 mg; placebo	9 years: 42.5% (0.2 DES, NS), 52% (1 DES, sign.), 43.8% (5 DES, sign.) vs. 50.6% (placebo)
VACURG II (M1) [40]	214	DES 0.2 mg; DES 1 mg; DES 5 mg; placebo	9 years: 30.8% (0.2 DES, NS), 43.6% (1 DES, sign.), 42.6% (5 DES, sign.) vs. 24.5% (placebo)
SAKK [4]	188	OX	19.2 vs. 19.55 (NS)
EORTC [5]	944	OX or LHRH	36.1 vs. 25% (sign.)

Study	n	Cancer-specific survival	Progression-free survival
Mayo	707	95 vs. 87% (sign.)	67 vs. 23% (sign.)
MRC	934	62 vs. 71% (sign.)	80.8 vs. 66.8% (sign.)
VACURG II (M0)	294	9 years: 87.6% (0.2 DES, NS), 59.9% (1 DES, sign.), 59.9 (5 DES, sign.) vs. 85.3% (placebo)	9 years: 42% (0.2 DES, NS), 82% (1 DES, sign.), 84% (5 DES, sign.) vs. 40% (placebo)
VACURG II (M1)	214	9 years: 46.2% (0.2 DES, NS), 69.1% (1 DES, sign.), 74 (5 DES, sign.) vs. 60.4% (placebo)	NA
SAKK	188	62 vs. 55% (NS)	42 vs. 20% (sign.)
EORTC	944	26 vs. 24.8% (NS)	41.8 vs. 30.5% (sign.)

RPX = radical prostatectomy; OX = oxaliplatin; LHRH = luteinizing hormone-releasing hormone; sign. = significant; NS = not significant; NA = not available.

nence for patients over 70. In contrast, three-dimensionally planned prostate radiotherapy becomes increasingly more important with advancing age. The risks and side effects of this therapy are low. In large series, lasting side effects of radiotherapy are found in only 3–5% of the cases. Incontinence is extremely rare [9]. The shorter follow-up times of radiotherapeutic procedures are of no consequence in relation to the likewise limited life expectancy. In this respect, the statement that the patient is unsuitable for curative therapy must be called into question.

Consequences of Progression

Advanced prostate cancer can cause the following 3 complications: (1) local infiltration, compression or displacement: subvesical obstruction, ureteric obstruction, rectal compression; (2) secondary complication through (osseous) metastases; (3) pain.

Pain and local progression can considerably impair the patient's quality of life. A spinal metastasis, for example, can lead to spinal cord compression or instability and thus to massive pain, sensory disturbances, pareses or dysfunction, or even paraplegia. If osseous metastases develop, life expectancy is also reduced in any case [10].

Uncertain Lymph Node Staging

Only surgical lymph node staging is suitable for a valid determination of lymph node status. Predicting the metastasis risk solely on the basis of tables such as the Partin Tables apparently often leads to false-negative results [11]. This is due to the fact that these tables were created on the basis of a lymph node dissection area limited only to the obturator fossa [12, 13]. If surgical staging is not performed at all in conjunction with delayed therapy, this important information is lacking. Patients with a positive lymph node status after radical prostatectomy had a markedly higher 10-year disease-specific survival if they received androgen deprivation therapy immediately after surgery than if hormone therapy was delayed until disease progression. The morbidity rate associated with spinal or ureteral compression was also reduced [14]. The patient's putatively reduced life expectancy must ultimately be weighed against the risk of inadequately treated lymph node metastases.

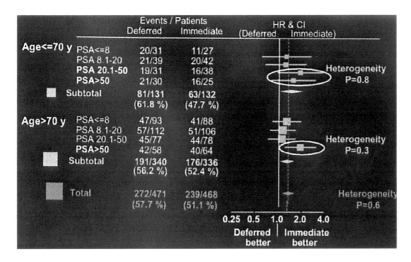

Fig. 1. EORTC 30891: total survival in the study according to initial PSA status and age at diagnosis [18].

Prostate-Specific Antigen as an Instrument of Control

Most studies examining the differences between immediate and deferred hormone deprivation therapy only initiate delayed treatment when symptomatic progression has developed. This could be the occurrence of painful metastases or local symptoms. The prostate-specific antigen (PSA) level has naturally only been considered in the most recent studies. This is due, on the one hand, to the fact that PSA was only widely adopted in urological practice in the 1980s. On the other hand, advocates of deferred therapy take the view that ultimately only symptoms require clinical consequences.

More recent studies use the PSA increase as an instrument of control. The fact that the surrogate parameter PSA strongly increases in most cases before symptoms develop is used here as an argument for initiating therapy to prevent grave consequences [15–17].

Extended assessment of the EORTC 30891 study suggests that the initial PSA should be used for risk estimation. Both progression-free and total survival showed particularly large differences, favoring immediate initiation in younger men (under 70) if the PSA was above 20 ng/ml at diagnosis and in older patients (over 70) if it was below 50 ng/ml (fig. 1 and 2) [18].

Besides the initial PSA value, the PSA velocity and doubling time are also particularly important for assessing tumor aggressiveness. Thus, patients with less favorable clinical stages and higher Gleason score sums have faster PSA doubling times [19]. In the follow-up of an active surveillance program, a PSA doubling time

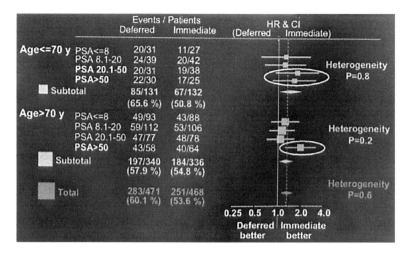

Fig. 2. EORTC 30891: progression-free survival according initial PSA status and age at diagnosis [18].

of less than 2 years is considered to be associated with a particularly poor prognosis. The optimal threshold value, below which therapy should be initiated, is around 3 years [17]. An analogous principle applies if biochemical recurrence develops after curative therapy, but here the prognostic cutoff of the doubling time is 3 months [20].

Hormone Deprivation Yesterday and Today

The side effects of surgical orchiectomy differ from those induced by DES. Particularly the probability of severe cardiovascular side effects is dramatically lower after an orchiectomy. Androgen deprivation is now commonly performed using a luteinizing hormone-releasing hormone (LHRH) analog with or without an additional testosterone receptor antagonist. The most frequent side effects are loss of libido, general tiredness and hot flushes; severe cases may also involve bone demineralization, fractures, muscular atrophy and metabolic disturbances [21–24]. According to various reports, the very stressful hot flushes must be expected more frequently under LHRH analog medication than after orchiectomy [25]. Patients in the above-mentioned studies had a median age of 75. Series examining the sexual life of prostate cancer patients in this age group show that on one hand, hormone ablation reduces or even abolishes potency, while on the other hand, this is a subjectively experienced problem in only very few patients [26]. In younger patients, however, the loss of potency is a much weightier component of the quality-of-life reduction.

From an economic viewpoint, no recognizable advantage can be gained by avoiding an orchiectomy. Compared to the considerable expenses arising from progression, such as from skeleton-related complications, heavy consequential costs are spared particularly by an orchiectomy, but also by using LHRH analogs.

Finally, it must be considered that hormone deprivation has a favorable effect on the subvesical obstruction very frequently seen in this age group. Apart from the cancer therapy, the patients are thus also denied a highly effective treatment of their micturition difficulties.

During the 50 years of experience with hormone deprivation in the treatment of prostate cancer, many highly effective concepts have been developed for preventing or treating possible side effects.

Erectile dysfunction – if this really poses a problem – can be treated by PDE5 inhibitors or corpus cavernosum autoinjection with prostaglandins [27]. If the therapy pause during intermittent hormone ablation is long enough for serum testosterone to regain its initial level, the patient can achieve temporary normalization of his sexual life with libido recovery [28, 29].

Hot flushes have often been successfully treated with megestrol acetate [30] or cyproterone acetate [31]. Gynecomastia can be prevented by prophylactic irradiation of the mammary glands [32]. Drug therapy can be considered with tamoxifen [33] or aromatase inhibitors [34]. Mostly only surgical measures are helpful if gland growth has already occurred. Osteoporosis can be successfully prevented or treated by administering zoledronic acid once a year [35, 36]. Calcium and vitamin D should also be supplemented [37].

Conclusion

More important than the issue of immediate versus deferred hormone deprivation therapy is the question of whether curative therapy is not (or no longer) possible. The long-term effect of radical prostatectomy or three-dimensionally planned radiotherapy surpasses that of hormone deprivation in many cases. Possible side effects are calculable, on the other hand. This must be carefully discussed with the patient.

If curative therapy really is unsuitable, the results of nearly all available studies indicate that immediate initiation of hormone therapy is best in terms of both total and progression-free survival. This applies particularly when the initial PSA is above 20 ng/ml in younger men (<70 years) and above 50 ng/ml in older patients (>70 years).

Considering the comorbidity and the tumor characteristics, particularly of the initial PSA, an individual risk analysis must be done and the patient must be clearly informed of the probable survival advantage gained by immediate therapy.

References

1 Huggins C, Hodges C: Studies on prostate cancer. I. The effect of estrogen and of androgen injection on serum phosphatases in metastatic carcinoma of the prostate. Cancer Res 1941;1:293–297.

2 Franksson C: Nobel Prize of the year. II. Charles B. Huggins. Lakartidningen 1966;63:4102–4104.

3 Blackard CE, Doe RP, Mellinger GT, Byar DP: Incidence of cardiovascular disease and death in patients receiving diethylstilbestrol for carcinoma of the prostate. Cancer 1970;26:249–256.

4 Studer UE, Hauri D, Hanselmann S, Chollet D, Leisinger HJ, Gasser T, Senn E, Trinkler FB, Tscholl RM, Thalmann GN, et al: Immediate versus deferred hormonal treatment for patients with prostate cancer who are not suitable for curative local treatment: results of the randomized trial SAKK 08/88. J Clin Oncol 2004;22:4109–4118.

5 Studer UE, Whelan P, Albrecht W, Casselman J, de Reijke T, Hauri D, Loidl W, Isorna S, Sundaram SK, Debois M, et al: Immediate or deferred androgen deprivation for patients with prostate cancer not suitable for local treatment with curative intent: European Organisation for Research and Treatment of Cancer (EORTC) Trial 30891. J Clin Oncol 2006;24:1868–1876.

6 Loblaw DA, Mendelson DS, Talcott JA, Virgo KS, Somerfield MR, Ben-Josef E, Middleton R, Porterfield H, Sharp SA, Smith TJ, et al: American Society of Clinical Oncology recommendations for the initial hormonal management of androgen-sensitive metastatic, recurrent, or progressive prostate cancer. J Clin Oncol 2004;22:2927–2941.

7 Nair B, Wilt T, MacDonald R, Rutks I: Early versus deferred androgen suppression in the treatment of advanced prostatic cancer. Cochrane Database Syst Rev 2002, Art No CD003506.

8 Tsevat J, Dawson NV, Wu AW, Lynn J, Soukup JR, Cook EF, Vidaillet H, Phillips RS: Health values of hospitalized patients 80 years or older. HELP Investigators. Hospitalized Elderly Longitudinal Project. JAMA 1998;279:371–375.

9 Pisansky TM: External-beam radiotherapy for localized prostate cancer. N Engl J Med 2006;355:1583–1591.

10 Soloway MS: The importance of prognostic factors in advanced prostate cancer. Cancer 1990;66:1017–1021.

11 Partin AW, Mangold LA, Lamm DM, Walsh PC, Epstein JI, Pearson JD: Contemporary update of prostate cancer staging nomograms (Partin Tables) for the new millennium. Urology 2001;58:843–848.

12 Bader P, Burkhard FC, Markwalder R, Studer UE: Is a limited lymph node dissection an adequate staging procedure for prostate cancer? J Urol 2002;168:514–518; discussion 518.

13 Heidenreich A, Varga Z, Von Knobloch R: Extended pelvic lymphadenectomy in patients undergoing radical prostatectomy: high incidence of lymph node metastasis. J Urol 2002;167:1681–1686.

14 Messing EM, Manola J, Yao J, Kiernan M, Crawford D, Wilding G, di'SantAgnese PA, Trump D: Immediate versus deferred androgen deprivation treatment in patients with node-positive prostate cancer after radical prostatectomy and pelvic lymphadenectomy. Lancet Oncol 2006;7:472–479.

15 Choo R, Klotz L, Danjoux C, Morton GC, DeBoer G, Szumacher E, Fleshner N, Bunting P, Hruby G: Feasibility study: watchful waiting for localized low to intermediate grade prostate carcinoma with selective delayed intervention based on prostate specific antigen, histological and/or clinical progression. J Urol 2002;167:1664–1669.

16 D'Amico AV, Moul JW, Carroll PR, Sun L, Lubeck D, Chen MH: Surrogate end point for prostate cancer-specific mortality after radical prostatectomy or radiation therapy. J Natl Cancer Inst 2003;95:1376–1383.

17 Klotz L: Active surveillance with selective delayed intervention using PSA doubling time for good risk prostate cancer. Eur Urol 2005;47:16–21.

18 Studer UE, Collette L, Whelan P, Albrecht W, Casselman J, De Reijke T, Hauri D, Loidl W, Isorna S, Sundaram SK: Patients with T0-4N0M0 Prostate Cancer not suitable for local treatment with curative intent (EORTC 30891): Which subgroup needs or does not need immediate treatment? J Urol 2006;175:1592.

19 Schmid HP, McNeal JE, Stamey TA: Observations on the doubling time of prostate cancer. The use of serial prostate-specific antigen in patients with untreated disease as a measure of increasing cancer volume. Cancer 1993;71:2031–2040.

20 D'Amico AV, Moul J, Carroll PR, Sun L, Lubeck D, Chen MH: Cancer-specific mortality after surgery or radiation for patients with clinically localized prostate cancer managed during the prostate-specific antigen era. J Clin Oncol 2003;21:2163–2172.

21 Daniell HW: Osteoporosis after orchiectomy for prostate cancer. J Urol 1997;157:439–444.

22 Townsend MF, Sanders WH, Northway RO, Graham SD Jr: Bone fractures associated with luteinizing hormone-releasing hormone agonists used in the treatment of prostate carcinoma. Cancer 1997;79:545–550.

23 Smith MR, Finkelstein JS, McGovern FJ, Zietman AL, Fallon MA, Schoenfeld DA, Kantoff PW: Changes in body composition during androgen deprivation therapy for prostate cancer. J Clin Endocrinol Metab 2002;87:599–603.

24 Herr HW, Kornblith AB, Ofman U: A comparison of the quality of life of patients with metastatic prostate cancer who received or did not receive hormonal therapy. Cancer 1993;71:1143–1150.

25 Karling P, Hammar M, Varenhorst E: Prevalence and duration of hot flushes after surgical or medical castration in men with prostatic carcinoma. J Urol 1994;152:1170–1173.

26 Potosky AL, Knopf K, Clegg LX, Albertsen PC, Stanford JL, Hamilton AS, Gilliland FD, Eley JW, Stephenson RA, Hoffman RM: Quality-of-life outcomes after primary androgen deprivation therapy: results from the Prostate Cancer Outcomes Study. J Clin Oncol 2001;19:3750–3757.

27 Kumar RJ, Barqawi A, Crawford ED: Preventing and treating the complications of hormone therapy. Curr Urol Rep 2005;6:217–223.

28 Kumar RJ, Barqawi A, Crawford ED: Adverse events associated with hormonal therapy for prostate cancer. Rev Urol 2005;7(suppl 5):S37–S43.

29 Bruchovsky N, Klotz LH, Sadar M, Crook JM, Hoffart D, Godwin L, Warkentin M, Gleave ME, Goldenberg SL: Intermittent androgen suppression for prostate cancer: Canadian Prospective Trial and related observations. Mol Urol 2000;4:191–199; discussion 201.

30 Loprinzi CL, Michalak JC, Quella SK, O'Fallon JR, Hatfield AK, Nelimark RA, Dose AM, Fischer T, Johnson C, Klatt NE, et al: Megestrol acetate for the prevention of hot flashes. N Engl J Med 1994;331:347–352.

31 Cervenakov I, Kopecny M, Jancar M, Chovan D, Mal'a M: 'Hot flush', an unpleasant symptom accompanying antiandrogen therapy of prostatic cancer and its treatment by cyproterone acetate. Int Urol Nephrol 2000;32:77–79.

32 Tyrrell CJ, Payne H, Tammela TL, Bakke A, Lodding P, Goedhals L, Van Erps P, Boon T, Van De Beek C, Andersson SO, et al: Prophylactic breast irradiation with a single dose of electron beam radiotherapy (10 Gy) significantly reduces the incidence of bicalutamide-induced gynecomastia. Int J Radiat Oncol Biol Phys 2004;60:476–483.

33 Serels S, Melman A: Tamoxifen as treatment for gynecomastia and mastodynia resulting from hormonal deprivation. J Urol 1998;159:1309.

34 Auclerc G, Antoine EC, Cajfinger F, Brunet-Pommeyrol A, Agazia C, Khayat D: Management of advanced prostate cancer. Oncologist 2000;5:36–44.

35 Simoneau AR: Treatment- and disease-related complications of prostate cancer. Rev Urol 2006;8(suppl 2):S56–S67.

36 Smith MR: Treatment-related osteoporosis in men with prostate cancer. Clin Cancer Res 2006;12:6315s–6319s.

37 Benton MJ, White A: Osteoporosis: recommendations for resistance exercise and supplementation with calcium and vitamin D to promote bone health. J Community Health Nurs 2006;23:201–211.

38 Zincke H, Lau W, Bergstralh E, Blute ML: Role of early adjuvant hormonal therapy after radical prostatectomy for prostate cancer. J Urol 2001;166:2208–2215.

39 Immediate versus deferred treatment for advanced prostatic cancer: initial results of the Medical Research Council Trial. The Medical Research Council Prostate Cancer Working Party Investigators Group. Br J Urol 1997;79:235–246.

40 Byar DP: Proceedings: The Veterans Administration Cooperative Urological Research Group's studies of cancer of the prostate. Cancer 1973;32:1126–1130.

PD Dr. M. Schostak
Department of Urology, Charité Universitätsmedizin Berlin, Campus Benjamin Franklin
Hindenburgdamm 30
DE–12200 Berlin (Germany)
Tel. +49 30 8445 2577, Fax +49 30 8445 4620, E-Mail martin.schostak@charite.de

Moser L, Schostak M, Miller K, Hinkelbein W (eds): Controversies in the Treatment of
Prostate Cancer. Front Radiat Ther Oncol. Basel, Karger, 2008, vol 41, pp 58–67

Lymphadenectomy in Prostate Cancer

Radio-Guided Lymph Node Mapping: An Adequate Staging Method

A. Winter   F. Wawroschek

Department of Urology, Klinikum Oldenburg, Oldenburg, Germany

Abstract

Lymph node status in prostate cancer is not only of prognostic but also of tremendous therapeutic relevance. In case of positive lymph nodes (N+), common standards demand the renunciation of local curative therapy (such as radiotherapy or radical prostatectomy) and hormonal withdrawal, or an appropriate adjuvant therapy can be planned (for example, early androgen ablation). But none of the currently available means of radiologic imaging (CT, MRT, PET-CT) provides sufficient identification of lymph node (micro)metastases (<5 mm). Also, predictive nomograms which are based on data from limited pelvic lymph node dissection (PLND) do not offer a sufficient grade of reliability. However, the limitation of the dissection area results in missing about 50–60% of N+ patients. In addition, the preoperative diagnostics often underestimate the true pathological stage. Presently, it seems that only the histological detection of lymph node metastases by methods with high sensitivity, like sentinel lymph node dissection or extended PLND, are suitable for lymph node staging in prostate cancer. The disadvantages of extended PLND are a high operative effort and increased complication rate. Therefore, sentinel lymph node dissection seems to strike a balance between high sensitivity and low complication rate.

Lymph node staging in prostate cancer has a significant clinical importance. Where the risk of progression can be calculated alternative appropriate adjuvant therapy can be planned. In case of positive lymph node (N+) findings, common standards demand the renunciation of local curative therapy (such as radical prostatectomy and radiotherapy) and hormonal withdrawal [1]. Moreover, there are studies which argue for early androgen ablation after radical prostatectomy in N+ patients [2]. Another opportunity is the modification of treatment volume in radiotherapy to optimize pelvic irradiation. The RTOG 94-13 trial has provided evidence that patients with high-risk prostate cancer benefit from additional irradiation to the pelvic nodes.

Statements regarding lymph node status in prostate cancer are based on radiologic imaging, predictive nomograms and surgical techniques of pelvic lymphadenectomy, including histopathological techniques of lymph node examination.

Radiologic Imaging

None of the currently available means of radiologic imaging provides sufficient identification of affected lymph nodes with a metastatic diameter of up to 5 mm. Computed tomography (CT) scans and magnetic resonance imaging (MRI) are routinely applied for primary diagnostics of lymph node metastases in prostate cancer. Positron emission tomography (PET) scans, PET-CT and radioimmunoscintigraphy are still limited to investigative studies.

CT scans and MRI are not able to identify lymph node metastases in the absence of nodal enlargement. However, the size of the nodes does not allow any sufficiently secure statement in terms of a benign or malignant nature. In a review of 25 studies (1,354 patients) on pelvic lymph node staging in clinically localized prostate cancer, no difference in the accuracy of CT and MRI (sensitivity 36%, specificity 97%) could be demonstrated. However, advances in MRI technology, like dynamic contrast-enhanced MRI or the development of a lymph node-specific contrast agent, are likely to increase its diagnostic value. It seems especially feasible to reduce the number of false-positive examinations. Nevertheless, ultrasmall superparamagnetic iron oxide particles have not yet been approved for diagnostics.

Radioimmunoscintigraphy using an indium-labeled antibody against prostate-specific membrane antigen (ProstaScint®) was not able to yield distinctively better results (sensitivity 44–75%, specificity 80–86%) than CT or MRI. A predictive value of only 66.7% was reached in a high-risk collective for lymph node metastases.

The same applied to PET using 2-desoxy-2-fluoro-D-glucose (FDG-PET) or 11C-acetate, in which a large number of small lymph node metastases remained undetected. A sensitivity of 30–75% and a specificity of 72–100% were described. Studies with fluorcholine PET-CT and C-11-choline PET-CT show a sensitivity of approximately 80% and a specificity of 95% [3].

Predictive Nomograms

The currently used predictive nomograms give the probability of nodal involvement for each individual patient based on preclinical data and multivariate analyses. The probability of lymph node metastases increases with the amount of prostate-specific antigen (PSA), the biopsy grade (Gleason score) and clinical T stage. But the preoperative diagnostics often underestimate the true pathological stage and grade. Understaging and undergrading are also a consequence of different biopsy techniques, too few biopsies and assessments by different pathologists. Furthermore, the nomograms are based on data from limited pelvic lymph node dissection (PLND) with a few lymph nodes being dissected.

The nomograms follow from large surgical series of pelvic lymphadenectomy and radical prostatectomy. The largest published series are those of Partin et al. [4], who analyzed the results of more than 4,000 patients in 3 institutions and over 5,000 patients in the nomogram update. For example, in the contemporary update of the Partin tables, the likelihood of lymph node metastases was 0–2% in men with PSA ≤10, biopsy Gleason score ≤6 and clinical stage ≤T2b (cancer in 1 lobe). Patients with clinical stage T2c and identical PSA and biopsy Gleason score had a 0–3% risk of lymphatic spread.

As a result of numerous nomograms, pelvic staging lymphadenectomy is no longer performed in patients with relatively favorable preoperative risk factors (PSA ≤10 ng/ml, Gleason score ≤7 and clinical stage ≤T2) in many centers. However, sentinel lymph node dissection (SLND) identifies N+ in patients with PSA ≤10 ng/ml and biopsy Gleason score ≤6 in 6.8% (positive biopsies in 1 lobe) and 10.7% (positive biopsies in both lobes) of patients [5].

Different Techniques of PLND

PLND is presently considered the gold standard for the identification of lymph node metastases in prostate cancer [1]. However, homogenous surgical standards concerning extent and technique of pelvic lymphadenectomy in prostate cancer cannot be gathered from the current literature. In relation to the intended therapy of prostate cancer (for example radiotheraphy, perineal or retropubic prostatectomy), pelvic lymphadenectomy can be carried out via different surgical accesses: laparotomy, minilaparotomy or laparoscopy.

The minimal variation – mostly carried out by means of laparoscopic pelvic lymphadenectomy – includes solely the lymphatic tissue of the so-called obturator fossa which is confined to the external iliac vein and to the obturator nerve. In contrast, Weingärtner et al. [6] concluded that about 20 lymph nodes must be dissected by means of the widespread standard of modified pelvic lymphadenectomy,

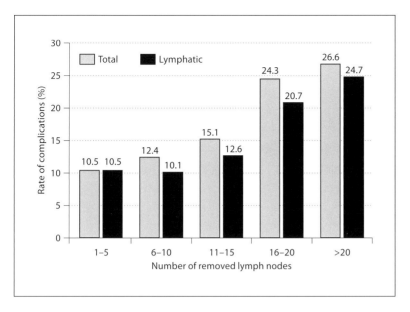

Fig. 1. Rate of complications dependent on the number of removed lymph nodes in PLND.

comprising lymphatic tissue surrounding the external iliac artery and vein, the obturator fossa and the obturator nerve. Others regard the resection of lymphatic tissue surrounding the common iliac artery, the external iliac artery and vein, the genitofemoral nerve, the obturator fossa as well as the region medial to the internal iliac artery surrounding its anterior arterial branches to be surgical standard (extended PLND) [7]. They describe the above-mentioned area of dissection minus the lymphatic tissue of common iliac artery and lateral to the external iliac artery as the so-called limited or modified PLND. The most current German variant of recommendation solely includes lymphatic tissue of the obturator fossa and surrounding the internal iliac artery [8].

The extended PLND has been shown to be associated with an increased risk of complications such as lymphocele, venous thrombosis, lower extremity edema and ureteral injury. Our own investigations [9] showed a significant increase in the complication rate – especially lymphatic complications – dependent on the number of resected lymph nodes: 1–5 lymph nodes: 10.5%; 6–10 lymph nodes: 12.4%; 11–15 lymph nodes: 15.1%; 16–20 lymph nodes: 24.3%; >20 lymph nodes: 26.6% (fig. 1). Authors who insist on a low complication rate of pelvic lymphadenectomy in most cases only have about 10 dissected lymph nodes in their specimens. Due to the high operative expenditure and the high morbidity related to extended PLND, the area of dissection has been reduced in most centers. But the systematic analysis of dissected lymph nodes deriving from complete PLND in

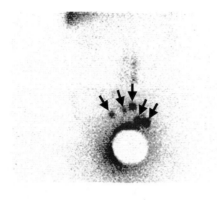

R V L   100'PI

Fig. 2. Scintigraphy of the prostate with 5 sentinel lymph nodes (arrows).

prostate cancer patients revealed that a reduction of the dissection area is problematic for the sensitivity of the detection of metastases [10, 11]. McDowell et al. [12] found isolated lymphatic spread in the presacral region and the tissue surrounding the vascular system of the internal iliac artery (superior and inferior vesical arteries, internal pudendal artery, hypogastric region) in 29% of patients with lymph node metastases. Limitation of the dissection area to the obturator fossa results in missing about 50–60% of the N+ patients [13].

Sentinel Concept in Prostate Cancer

Because of the above-mentioned difficulties of extended (high morbidity) and limited PLND (low sensitivity), SLND was educed for selective dissection of the primarily draining lymph nodes of the prostate. Studies which were restricted to the scintigraphic representation of the lymphatic drainage region of the prostate formed the basis for the introduction of the sentinel lymph node concept in prostate carcinoma. The identification of sentinel lymph nodes in prostate cancer is in principle different from the technique in other tumor entities. For example, in breast cancer, penis cancer as well as in malignant melanoma, a well-directed peritumoral injection is placed only to observe the lymphatic drainage of the tumor. In prostate cancer, however, it is not known from which part of the organ the metastatic spread originates. Therefore, the aim of prostate lymphoscintigraphy (fig. 2) has to be the imaging of all primarily draining lymph nodes of the prostate, which inevitably include the sentinel lymph nodes of the tumor.

In 1998, scintigraphy combined with intraoperative detection via gamma probe was applied for the first time to prove sentinel node presence [14]. In the following years, radio-guided surgery was established in prostate cancer by many groups. Until now, more than 1,000 patients have been evaluated [13, 15].

For sentinel lymph node detection, ^{99m}Tc-nanocolloid [13], ^{99m}Tc-rhenium sulphur colloid [16] or phytate [17] are used. Probably, the new tracer Lymphoseek (^{99m}Tc-diethylenetetramine pentaacetic acid-mannosyl-dextran) offers a new opportunity for direct intraoperative injection [18]. Wide experience exists with ^{99m}Tc-nanocolloid. The tracer is applied transrectally into the prostate under ultrasound guidance the day before lymphadenectomy. For preoperative visualization of sentinel lymph nodes, lymphoscintigraphies are performed in different intervals after injection. Alternatively, single photon emission CT (SPECT) or SPECT/CT fusion imaging can be used. Intraoperatively, the sentinel lymph nodes are detected by gamma probe.

The evaluation of our collective resulted in 21.1% N+ cases [19]. The analysis of 860 patients with SLND showed only 2 falsely negative patients. Thus, the sensitivity was >97%. In contrast, we demonstrated a sensitivity of just 79.2% [5] for the modified PLND. Metastases were often exclusively located in the hypogastric region, a region which is not included in the modified (standard) PLND. More than 60% of the N+ patients would have been falsely classified as pN0 stage if only a standard PLND had been done. The results of extended PLND are certified herewith [11].

Histopathological Examination and Influence on the Detection Rate of N+ Patients

It is not only the extent of pelvic lymphadenectomy that has a significant influence on lymph node status in prostate cancer, but also the nature of the histopathological examination (step sections, serial section, immunohistochemistry and RT-PCR).

Extended histopathological technique (step sections, serial sections and immunohistochemistry) could reach a diagnostic improvement of about 14% [20]. For example, by using conventional histological technique, lymph node metastases were found in 5% of patients with preoperative PSA <10 ng/ml, clinical stage T2 and Gleason score in biopsy <7. By adding serial sections, metastases were found in 11.3%.

The PSA-specific RT-PCR is a new and revealing supplementary technique for the detection of tumor cells in sentinel lymph nodes of prostate cancer patients. Haas et al. [21] showed that 4 of 12 patients with biochemical relapse, but without positive margins or (immuno)histological N+, were RT-PCR positive for PSA.

Limitations of SLND in Prostate Cancer

Prostate lymphoscintigraphy seemed to be influenced by a neoadjuvant hormonal therapy provided over a long period of time (>3 months). This might also be the cause of the low number of sentinel lymph nodes (70.8%) in the investigation by Takashima et al. [17], in which 75% of the patients were treated with hormonal deprivation. Also, a previous transurethral resection or transvesical surgery of the prostate leads to postoperative alterations in lymphatic drainage. Macrometastases or tumor deposits which obstruct lymphatic vessels might also be a problem and can lead to false-negative results. However, macrometastases in patients with clinically localized prostate cancer are extremely rare.

Is There a Potential Therapeutic Benefit of PLND in Prostate Cancer?

Presently it is unclear whether N+ patients will have a better prediction after removing diseased nodes. However, a few studies showed a potential therapeutic benefit of PLND in prostate cancer.

According to data published by Catalona et al. [22], one can suggest lymphadenectomy as a therapeutic measure. In a small collective, 75% of patients (total 12) with lymph node metastases and no adjuvant therapy remained without biochemical relapse at 6 years, and 58% after 7 years. Bader et al. [23] showed that the number of lymph node metastases detected strictly correlates with the number of removed nodes, and that the rate of pN0 patients with tumor progression is higher in those with only few nodes removed. Also, they showed that 38.5% of patients with only 1 N+, 10% with 2 and 14% with more N+ remained disease free after 45 months (median). In another study, N+ patients had a progression-free survival of 70% (1 N+) or 73% (2 N+) after 10 years [24]. The PSA progression-free survival could improve especially in N+ patients with low-risk prostate cancer (PSA ≤ 10 ng/ml, Gleason score ≤ 6). Weckermann et al. [25] demonstrated that 60% of the patients with N+ and no hormone therapy (total 25) remained relapse free after a follow-up of 18 months.

Relevance of Sentinel Concept for Radiotherapy of Prostate Cancer

Patients with high-risk disease seem to benefit from an additional radiotherapy to the pelvic lymph nodes combined with hormonal ablation (RTOG 94-13 trial). Because of the high variability of lymphatic drainage, the sentinel concept offers an option to optimize the target volume for the pelvic lymph nodes. Ganswindt et al. [26] reported that intensity-modulated radiotherapy based on sentinel lymph node identification by SPECT is feasible and allows a pronounced sparing of normal tissue irradiation.

Conclusions

PLND seems to be presently indispensable for exact lymph node staging in prostate cancer due to the inadequacy of alternative nonoperative techniques for the identification of lymph node micrometastases. However, homogeneous surgical standards for PLND for prostate cancer do not exist at present. Because of the high morbidity and effort of extended PLND, most centers have decreased the area of dissection. But any limitation of the dissection area corresponds with a reduced detection rate of micrometastases. The widespread limitation of the dissection area to the so-called obturator fossa lymph nodes results in missing about 50% of N+ patients.

Radio-guided lymph node dissection considers the interindividual variance of prostatic lymph drainage. SLND offers a reduced time of resection and lower morbidity in comparison to the extended forms of pelvic lymphadenectomy, without having to expect a significantly reduced detection of micrometastases.

In contrast to the clinical algorithms, which provide statistical probabilities for populations of patients with similar clinical variables, pelvic lymphadenectomy renders a precise lymph node staging and a potential benefit regarding progression of disease for the individual patient. It has been clearly demonstrated that more patients than previously believed are bearing micrometastasis in particular, also in the case of clinically localized prostate cancer.

As a consequence, lymph node surgery including the primary lymph nodes of the prostate is essential for most patients before or during therapy with curative intent (radiotherapy and prostatectomy). This might not only be of prognostic relevance for the patient, but also have a therapeutic background. Data from centers which perform extended PLND or SLND in case of radical prostatectomy demonstrate that patients with singular lymph node metastasis are possibly free of PSA recurrence in long-term follow-ups. In this regard, a combination of SLND and extended PLND in patients with high-risk prostate cancer could make sense if one is positive about a better survival by removal of the fourth or fifth lymph node metastasis.

References

1 Aus G, Abbou CC, Bolla M, Heidenreich A, Schmid HP, van Poppel H, Wolff J, Zattoni F: EAU guidelines on prostate cancer. Eur Urol 2005;48:546–551.

2 Messing EM, Manola J, Sarosdy M, Wilding G, Crawford ED, Trump D: Immediate hormonal therapy compared with observation after radical prostatectomy and pelvic lymphadenectomy in men with node positive prostate cancer: results at 10 years of EST 3886. J Urol 2003;169(suppl 4): 396.

3 Seitz M, Khoder W, Schlenker B, Gratzke C, Reich O, Stief C: Klinische Relevanz der 11C-Cholin PET/CT beim Prostatakarzinom. Urologe 2006;45(suppl 1):102.

4 Partin AW, Mangold LA, Lamm DM, Walsh PC, Epstein JI, Pearson JD: Contemporary update of prostate cancer staging nomograms (Partin Tables) for the new millennium. J Urol 2001;58: 843–848.

5 Weckermann D, Wawroschek F, Harzmann R: Is there a need for pelvic lymph node dissection in low risk prostate cancer patients prior to definitive local therapy? Eur Urol 2005;47:45–51.

6 Weingärtner K, Ramaswamy A, Bittinger A, Gerharz EW, Voge D, Riedmiller H: Anatomical basis for pelvic lymphadenectomy in prostate cancer: results of an autopsy study and implications for the clinic. J Urol 1996;156:1969–1971.

7 Schuessler WW, Pharand D, Vancaille TG: Laparosopic standard pelvic node dissection for carcinoma of the prostate: is it accurate? Urology 1993; 150:898–901.

8 Leitlinien zur Diagnostik von Prostatakarzinomen. Mitteilungen der DGU und des BDU. Urologe A 1999;38:388–401.

9 Winter A, Vogt C, Weckermann D, Harzmann R, Wawroschek F: Komplikationsraten verschiedener LA-Techniken beim klinisch lokalisierten Prostatakarzinom im Vergleich. Urologe 2005; 44(suppl 1):79.

10 Heidenreich A, Varga Z, von Knobloch R: Extended pelvic lymphadenectomy in patients undergoing radical prostatectomy: high incidence of lymph node metastasis. J Urol 2002;167:1681–1686.

11 Bader P, Burkhard FC, Markwalder R, Studer UE: Is a limited lymph node dissection an adequate staging procedure for prostate cancer? J Urol 2002;168:514–518.

12 McDowell GC, Johnson JW, Tenney DM, Johnson DE: Pelvic lymphadenectomy for staging clinically localized prostate cancer: indications, complications, and results in 217 cases. Urology 1990;35:476–482.

13 Wawroschek F, Vogt H, Wengenmair, Hamm M, Keil M, Graf G, Heidenreich P, Harzmann R: Prostate lymphoscintigraphy and radio-guided surgery for sentinel lymph node identification in prostate cancer: technique and results of the first 350 cases. Urol Int 2003;70:303–310.

14 Wawroschek F, Vogt H, Weckermann D, Wagner T, Hamm M, Harzmann R: Radioisotope-guided pelvic lymph node dissection for prostate cancer. J Urol 2001;166:1715–1719.

15 Goppelt M, Holl G, Wagner T, Harzmann R, Weckermann D: Sentinellymphadenectomy beim Prostatakarzinom: Erfahrungen nach über 1,000 Fällen. Urologe 2006;45(suppl 1):102–103.

16 Silva N Jr, Anselmi CE, Anselmi OE, Madke RR, Hunsche A, Souto JS, Souto CA, Sica FD, Pioner GT, Macalos EC, Hartmann A A, Lima MS: Use of gamma probe in sentinel lymph node biopsy in patients with prostate cancer. Nucl Med Commun 2005;26:1081–1086.

17 Takashima H, Egawa M, Imao T, Fukuda M, Yokoyama K, Namika M: Validity of sentinel lymph node concept for patients with prostate cancer. J Urol 2004;171:2268–2271.

18 Salem CE, Hoh CK, Wallace A M, Vera DR: A preclinical study of prostate sentinel lymph node mapping with [^{99M}TC]diethylenetetramine pentaacetic acid-mannosyl-dextran. J Urol 2006;175: 44–48.

19 Weckermann D, Hamm M, Dorn R, Wagner T, Wawroschek F, Harzmann R: Sentinel lymph node dissection in prostate cancer: experience after more than 800 interventions. Urologe 2006; 45:723–727.

20 Wawroschek F, Wagner T, Hamm M, Weckermann D, Vogt H, Märkl B, Gordijn R, Harzmann R: The influence of serial sections, immunohistochemistry, and extension of pelvic lymph node dissection on the lymph node status in clinically localized prostate cancer. Eur Urol 2003;43:132–137.

21 Haas J, Wagner T, Wawroschek F, Arnold H: Combined application of RT-PCR and immuno-histochemistry on paraffin embedded sentinel lymph nodes of prostate cancer patients. Pathol Res Pract 2005;200:763–770.

22 Catalona WJ, Miller DR, Kavoussi LR: Intermediate-term survival results in clinically under-
stated prostate cancer patients following radical
prostatectomy. J Urol 1988;140:540–543.

23 Bader P, Burkhard FC, Markwalder R, Studer UE:
Disease progression and survival of patients with
positive lymph nodes after radical prostatectomy. Is there a chance of cure? J Urol 2003;169:
849–854.

24 Daneshmand S, Quek ML, Stein JP, Lieskovsky
G, Cai J, Pinski J, Skinner EC, Skinner DG:
Prognosis of patients with lymph node positive
prostate cancer following radical prostatectomy: long-term results. J Urol 2004;172:2252–
2255.

25 Weckermann D, Goppelt M, Dorn R, Wawroschek F, Harzmann R: Incidence of positive pelvic lymph nodes in patients with prostate cancer,
a prostate-specific antigen (PSA) level of ≤ 10 ng/
ml and biopsy Gleason score of ≤ 6, and their influence on PSA progression-free survival after
radical prostatectomy. BJU Int. 2006;97:1173–
1178.

26 Ganswindt U, Paulsen F, Corvin S, Eichhorn K,
Glocker S, Hundt I, Birkner M, Alber M, Anas-
tasiadis A, Stenzl A, Bares R, Budach W, Bamberg
M, Belka C: Intensity modulated radiotherapy for
high risk prostate cancer based on sentinel node
SPECT imaging for target volume definition.
BMC Cancer 2005;5:91.

Dr. Alexander Winter
Department of Urology, Klinikum Oldenburg
Dr.-Eden-Strasse 10
DE–26133 Oldenburg (Germany)
Tel. +49 441 4032 302, Fax +49 441 4032 303, E-Mail winter.alexander@klinikum-oldenburg.de

Moser L, Schostak M, Miller K, Hinkelbein W (eds): Controversies in the Treatment of
Prostate Cancer. Front Radiat Ther Oncol. Basel, Karger, 2008, vol 41, pp 68–76

Radiotherapy in Lymph Node-Positive Prostate Cancer Patients – A Potential Cure?

Single Institutional Experience Regarding Outcome and Side Effects

Gregor Goldner   Richard Pötter

Department of Radiotherapy and Radiobiology, Medical School, University of Vienna,
Vienna, Austria

Abstract

Some studies have shown that a number of patients with positive lymph nodes may be potentially curable. Seventy-five lymph node-positive prostate cancer patients were treated by radiotherapy alone (36%) or by radiotherapy after radical prostatectomy (64%). The prostatic region was irradiated in 20 patients (27%) and the prostatic region plus pelvic lymph nodes in 55 (73%). The median lymph node dose was 46 Gy, the median dose at the prostatic region 67 Gy. Biochemical no evidence of disease (bNED), overall survival as well as acute/late gastrointestinal and urogenital side effects were evaluated. Median follow-up was 40 months (range 1–132). Five- and eight-year bNED rates were 54% and 51%, respectively; 5- and 8-year overall survival rates were 78% and 67%, respectively. Concerning bNED and overall survival, no significant difference in regard to treatment technique (prostatic region vs. prostatic region plus pelvic lymph nodes) or treatment strategy (radical prostatectomy plus radiotherapy vs. radiotherapy alone) was found. Four of seventy-five patients showed no prostate-specific antigen progression after 9 years. Acute/late gastrointestinal and urogenital side effects were mostly moderate, revealing no difference in severity regarding treatment technique. To conclude, advanced treatment techniques allowing dose escalation in the prostatic and pelvic region should be considered in selected lymph node-positive prostate cancer patients in order to further improve clinical outcome.

Patients presenting with lymph node-positive prostate cancer at diagnosis have an increased risk of distant metastases and therefore have a relatively poor prognosis if a single treatment modality such as radiotherapy, surgery or hormonal therapy is applied. Independent from surgery or radiotherapy as the selected treatment, only 20–30% of patients will survive at 10 years [1–3]. Hanks et al. [3] reported about 29% overall survival (OS) and 7% clinical cancer-free survival 10 years after primary radiotherapy alone. Radiotherapy combined with early hormonal therapy was able to improve survival. Wiegel and Bressel [4] reported a 10-year survival of 45% after radiotherapy and orchiectomy. Sands et al. [5] showed that combined local radiotherapy and early androgen ablation significantly improved clinical response compared to patients treated with early androgen ablation alone. Some studies have shown that the number of involved lymph nodes and the extent of nodal involvement are important prognostic factors [4–6]. Therefore, a significant number of patients with positive lymph nodes that may be selected at diagnosis may be potentially curable or will at least achieve long-time remission beyond 10 years.

However, there has been only moderate development regarding radiotherapy within the last decades for treating lymph node-positive prostate cancer patients. Advanced techniques allowing dose escalation are limited in general to localized prostate cancer patients.

Patients and Methods

Patients
Seventy-five patients with histologically proven prostate cancer and positive lymph nodes (T1–4N1M0/1) – verified by either lymphadenectomy or computed tomography (CT) – underwent three-dimensional conformal radiotherapy between January 1995 and March 2006. To detect distant metastasis, a bone scan in patients presenting with prostate-specific antigen (PSA) >30 ng/ml at diagnosis was performed. The treatment procedure included an initial radical prostatectomy followed by radiotherapy or primary radiotherapy combined with additional hormonal therapy.

Radiation Technique
All patients were treated in supine position by the 4-field box technique (25×10^6 V photons) with individualized blocks derived from beam's eye view. The clinical target volume was defined based on series of CT and included the prostatic region with or without the pelvic lymph nodes. The planning target volume included a margin of 0.5–1.2 cm for the prostatic region and 1.0–1.5 cm for the pelvic lymph nodes. Radiation dose was specified at the ICRU reference point.

Follow-Up
Acute gastrointestinal (aGI) and urogenital (aUG) side effects were documented prospectively by use of the EORTC/RTOG score before, during (first, second and third third of radiation) and 6 weeks after radiotherapy.

All measures of time were calculated from the last day of radiotherapy. During the first 2 years after radiotherapy, patients were seen every 3–6 months and at least once a year thereafter. Follow-up included a complete history, physical examination, transrectal ultrasound and serum PSA. Late gastrointestinal (GI) and urogenital (UG) side effects were scored prospectively according to the EORTC/RTOG criteria. Biochemical no evidence of disease (bNED) was defined according to the ASTRO guidelines as 3 consecutive rises in serum PSA [7].

Statistical Analysis
Data were analyzed using SPSS® statistical software. A value of $p < 0.05$ was considered significant. Survival times were calculated by the Kaplan-Meier method using the log-rank test for univariate analysis. The influence of T stage, grading/Gleason score, maximal pretreatment PSA, hormonal therapy (yes/no), distant metastasis (yes/no), intention to treat (radical prostatectomy plus radiotherapy/radiotherapy) and treatment technique (prostatic region alone/prostatic region plus pelvic lymph node irradiation) on bNED and OS was investigated by Cox regressions for multivariate analysis.

Results

Patients
The median follow-up was 40 months (range 1–132). The median age was 67 years (range 49–91). Positive lymph nodes were verified by lymphadenectomy in 23 patients (30%) and by CT in 52 (70%) The distribution of patients with versus without lymph node irradiation was 55 (73%) versus 20 patients (27%). The median lymph node dose was 46 Gy (range 36–55) and the median dose for all patients at the prostatic region was 67 Gy (range 46–74).

An initial radical prostatectomy followed by radiotherapy was performed in 27 patients (36%). Of these, 20 (74%) also received hormonal treatment. Primary radiotherapy was performed in 48 patients (64%). All of these patients received hormonal therapy.

The patients' distributions concerning T stage, histological grading, maximal pretreatment PSA, distant metastasis, additional hormonal therapy and radiation technique are shown in detail in table 1.

Side Effects
The data on the maximum cumulative aGI/aUG toxicity, which was mostly low to moderate, are available for all 75 patients. Grade 0 and 1 were seen for aGI side effects in 52/75 patients (69%) and for aUG side effects in 58/75 (77%), respectively. Grade 2 aGI side effects were found in 23/75 patients (31%) and Grade 2 aUG side effects in 17/75 (23%).

Concerning late GI/UG side effects, the data are available for 72/75 patients (96%) with a median follow-up of 40 months. Late GI side effects were mostly low to moderate with Grade 0 and 1 in 63/72 patients (88%). Grade 2 and 3 GI side effects were found in 7 and 2 patients (10 and 3%), respectively. Late UG side effects of grade 0 or 1, 2 and 3 were seen in 60 (83%), 10 (14%) and 2 patients (3%), respectively. Table 2 shows the distribution of grade ≥ 2 acute and late side effects in regard to treatment technique without finding a significant difference between patients treated at the prostatic region alone compared to patients treated with additional lymph node irradiation. Similarly, the actuarial rate of late side effects of grade ≥ 2 showed no significant difference (fig. 1a, b).

Table 1. Patient characteristics

	Prostatic region (n = 20)	Prostatic region + pelvic lymph nodes (n = 55)	Total (n = 75)
Tumor stage			
T1	–	3 (5)	3 (4)
T2	5 (25)	10 (18)	15 (20)
T3	11 (55)	31 (56)	42 (56)
T4	4 (20)	11 (20)	15 (20)
Grading/Gleason score			
1/2–3	1 (5)	3 (5)	4 (5)
2/4–6	4 (20)	15 (27)	19 (25)
3/7–10	15 (75)	33 (60)	48 (65)
G x	–	4 (7)	4 (5)
Maximal initial PSA			
<20 ng/ml	9 (45)	21 (38)	30 (40)
20–50 ng/ml	6 (30)	14 (25)	20 (27)
>50 ng/ml	5 (25)	20 (36)	25 (33)
Distant metastasis	3 (15)	5 (9)	8 (11)
Hormonal therapy	17 (85)	51 (93)	68 (91)
Radiation technique			
Radiotherapy	10 (50)	17 (31)	27 (36)
RPE + radiotherapy	10 (50)	38 (69)	48 (64)
Dose at prostatic region, Gy[1]	66.2 (60–74)	67.9 (46.4–73)	
Dose at pelvic region, Gy[1]	–	46 (36–55)	

Figures in parentheses are percentages, unless indicated otherwise. G x = unknown; RPE = radical prostatectomy.
[1] Figures in parentheses are ranges.

Table 2. Distribution of grade ≥2 acute and late GI and UG side effects in regard to treatment procedure

	Acute GI	Acute UG	Late GI	Late UG
Prostatic region, %	35	25	15	20
Prostatic region + pelvic LN, %	29	22	11	15

LN = Lymph node.

Disease Control

The 5-year/8-year bNED and OS rates for all patients were 54/51% and 78/67%, respectively. Figure 2 shows bNED and OS rates for patients treated within the prostatic region compared to patients treated at the prostatic region plus pelvic

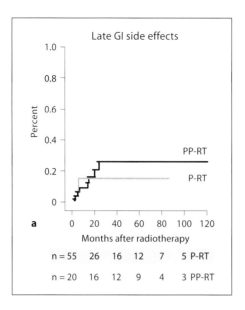
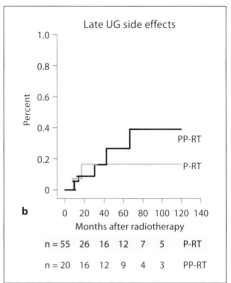

Fig. 1. a Late GI side effects grade ≥2 (EORTC/RTOG): prostatic irradiation versus prostatic and pelvic irradiation (p = 0.7). **b** Late UG side effects grade ≥2 (EORTC/RTOG): prostatic irradiation versus prostatic and pelvic irradiation (p = 0.7). PP-RT = Prostatic + pelvic irradiation; P-RT = prostatic irradiation.

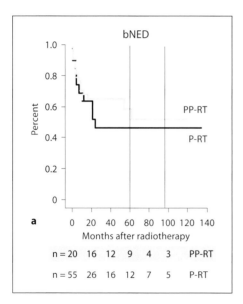
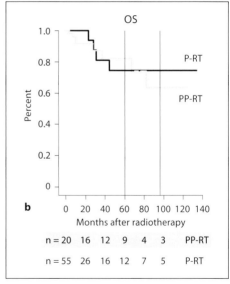

Fig. 2. a bNED survival for patients with prostatic irradiation (5 years: 46%; 8 years: 46%) versus patients with prostatic and pelvic irradiation (5 years: 58%; 8years: 52%) without any significant difference (p = 0.5). **b** OS for patients with prostatic irradiation (5 years: 74%; 8 years: 74%) versus patients with prostatic and pelvic irradiation (5 years: 82%; 8 years: 63%) without any significant difference (p = 0.8). PP-RT = Prostatic + pelvic irradiation; P-RT = prostatic irradiation.

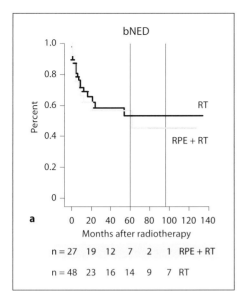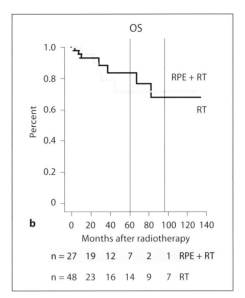

Fig. 3. a bNED survival for patients after radical prostatectomy and radiotherapy (5 years: 56%; 8 years: 45%) versus patients with radiotherapy alone (5 years: 53%; 8 years: 53%) without any significant difference (p = 0.7). **b** OS for patients after radical prostatectomy and radiotherapy (5 years: 71%; 8 years: 71%) versus patients with radiotherapy alone (5 years: 83%; 8 years: 68%) without any significant difference (p = 0.8). RPE + RT = Radical prostatectomy and radiotherapy; RT = radiotherapy.

lymph nodes, without finding a significant difference. Figure 3a and b shows bNED and OS rates regarding treatment strategy by comparing patients treated with radical prostatectomy plus radiotherapy to patients treated by radiotherapy alone, again without finding a significant difference.

In multivariate analysis, only pretreatment PSA (p = 0.007) and distant metastasis (p = 0.02) were found to be significant factors influencing bNED. In regard to OS, no significant factor was found performing multivariate analysis.

Discussion

The number of studies dealing with the radiotherapy of lymph node-positive prostate cancer patients is limited. However, some patient- and treatment-related factors, such as number of positive lymph nodes, extent of lymph node invasion and additional hormonal therapy, influencing clinical outcome have been reported [3–6].

An optimal treatment procedure of lymph node-positive prostate cancer patients has not yet been determined. Independent from surgery or radiotherapy as the selected treatment, only 20–30% of patients will survive at 10 years due to the

Table 3. Characteristics of 9-year bNED patients

Follow-up, months	T stage	Grade	N+ diagnosis	N+ nodes, n	HT	Treat-ment	RT technique	PSA level
119	4	1	LND	2	yes	RT only	+ pelvic	0.04
118	2	2	LND	1	yes	RT only	+ pelvic	0.51
108	3	3	CT	1 (2 cm)	yes	RT only	+ pelvic	0.05
132	3	2	LND	1	yes	RT only	local	0.26

N+ = Positive lymph node; HT = hormonal therapy; RT = radiation; LND = lymph node dissection.
Radiation technique: 46 Gy pelvic; 66 Gy prostate.

high risk of distant metastasis [1–3]. Hormonal therapy alone will produce resistant clones, resulting within a certain time period in a high risk also of local recurrence [8]. The combination of local treatment (surgery or radiotherapy) and systemic treatment (adjuvant hormonal therapy) is therefore regarded as the treatment of choice.

Whittington et al. [9] reported a 6-year survival rate of 82% in 50 lymph node-positive patients treated with combined hormonal and radiation therapy. All patients received pelvic radiation to 45 Gy, with a boost dose to the prostate to 65–71 Gy. Forty-five patients were treated with radiotherapy plus hormonal therapy and 5 patients with radiotherapy alone. Of these 5 patients, only 1 survived longer than 3 years. They concluded that the combination of radiotherapy and hormonal therapy was effective for lymph node-positive prostate cancer patients.

Sands et al. [5] reported 27 lymph node-positive patients receiving hormonal therapy and radiation with a pelvic dose up to 46 Gy and a prostatic dose up to 66 Gy. They compared this group to 181 patients treated by hormonal therapy alone and showed that combined local radiotherapy and early androgen ablation significantly improved clinical response. At 4 years, 45% of patients in the hormonal therapy only group versus 100% of patients in the radiotherapy/hormonal therapy group showed no signs of rising PSA or progression (p = 0.002).

For the RTOG 75-06 protocol, Hanks et al. [3] reported 90 patients with biopsy-proven positive lymph nodes treated with radiotherapy alone. The 5-year/10-year survival was 63/29% and the 5-year/10-year clinical disease-free survival was 32/7%. They found a small fraction (2/90) of node-positive prostate cancer patients to be cured of their disease at 10 years after radiotherapy. Similar to Hanks et al. [3], we also found a small number of patients (4/75 patients) without any evidence of PSA progression presenting with a follow-up of at least 9 years. Table 3 shows the details of these patients in regard to follow-up, stage, grading, diagnosis of lymph nodes, hormonal therapy, treatment, radiation technique and current PSA value.

The number of positive lymph nodes at diagnosis is important. Hanks et al. [3] found only patients presenting with 1 or 2 positive nodes (2 of 39 patients) to be cured. Gervasi et al. [6] reported the results of 152 patients treated with radiotherapy and hormonal therapy. They found a significantly better 10-year survival in patients with solitary lymph node involvement compared to multiple involved nodes (60 vs. 37%). Similar to these results, the number of positive lymph nodes in our long-time relapse-free survivors was only 1 or 2.

Wiegel and Bressel [4] reported about 70 node-positive patients treated with pelvic irradiation up to 40–50 Gy and boost to the prostatic region in 67/70 patients to deliver 60–70 Gy. Prior to radiotherapy, 30 patients initially had a radical prostatectomy with orchiectomy and 40 patients had only an orchiectomy. With a median follow-up of 58 months, the OS rate at 5 and 10 years was 78 and 45%, respectively.

Our 5- and 8-year survival rates were 78 and 67%, respectively. Similar to Wiegel and Bressel [4], our patients were also treated by radical prostatectomy and radiotherapy (64%) or radiotherapy alone (36%). Taking into account the shorter follow-up of 40 months in our study, these data are in good agreement.

There has been only moderate development regarding radiotherapy within the last decades for treating node-positive prostate cancer patients. The risk of developing significant late GI and UG side effects is considered to limit the radiation dose needed for treating pelvic lymph nodes efficiently. Roach et al. [10] analyzed the incidence of late side effects in patients treated with prostate-only radiotherapy (PO, 131 patients) and whole-pelvis radiotherapy (WP, 309 patients). In this RTOG 94-13 protocol, patients were treated by radiotherapy without the use of three-dimensional treatment planning and showed a significant increase in toxicity. Grade ≥ 2 late GI side effects were 15.2% (WP) versus 7.0% (PO) and grade ≥ 2 late UG side effects were 14.9% (WP) versus 5.6% (PO).

By the use of three-dimensional treatment planning, the incidence of side effects can be reduced. In our analysis of 75 patients, no increase in toxicity was found when pelvic radiotherapy with additional boost to the prostatic region was performed. The amount of maximal acute as well as grade ≥ 2 late GI and UG side effects showed no significant difference (table 2) and also the actuarial rates of grade ≥ 2 late side effects were not found to differ significantly (fig. 1a and b). One limitation of this retrospective analysis is the small number of patients. However, by comparing prostate (n >900) versus pelvic radiation (n >150) of all prostate cancer patients evaluated at our institution treated from 1994 to 2006, we could again find no significant difference in regard to late GI and UG side effects [unpubl. data].

Patients presenting with positive lymph nodes at diagnosis are good candidates for innovative treatment approaches, as advanced treatment techniques like intensity-modulated radiotherapy and image-guided radiotherapy have the potential to increase pelvic radiation dose to 60 Gy without significantly increasing the incidence of acute and late side effects.

Conclusion

Only about 50% of our patients show bNED at 5 years after treatment. The number of patients without any signs of PSA progression presenting with a follow-up of at least 9 years is small. Advanced treatment techniques should therefore be considered for lymph node-positive prostate cancer patients in order to increase the amount of pelvic control, and consequently the number of long-time survivors, without increasing treatment-related morbidity.

References

1 DeKernion JB, Neuwirth H, Stein A, Dorey F, Stenzl A, Hannah J, Blyth B: Prognosis of patients with stage D1 prostate carcinoma following radical prostatectomy with and without early endocrine therapy. J Urol 1990;144:700–703.

2 Steinberg GD, Epstein JI, Piantadosi S, Walsh PC: Management of stage D1 adenocarcinoma of the prostate: the Johns Hopkins experience 1974–1987. J Urol 1990;144:1425–1432.

3 Hanks GE, Buzydlowski J, Sause WT, Emami B, Rubin P, Parsons JA, Russell AH, Byhardt RW, Earle JD, Pilepich MV: Ten-year outcomes for pathologic node-positive patients treated in RTOG 75-06. Int J Radiat Oncol Biol Phys 1998;40:765–768.

4 Wiegel T, Bressel M: Influence of the extent of nodal involvement on the outcome in stage D1 prostate cancer. Radiat Oncol Invest 1994;2:144–151.

5 Sands E, Pollack A, Zagars GK: Influence of radiotherapy on node-positive prostate cancer treated with androgen ablation. Int J Radiat Oncol Biol Phys 1995;31:13–19.

6 Gervasi LA, Mata J, Easley JD, Wilbanks JH, Seale-Hawkins C, Carlton CE Jr, Scardino PT: Prognostic significance of lymph nodal metastases in prostate cancer. J Urol 1989;142:332–336.

7 Consensus statement: guidelines for PSA following radiation therapy. American Society for Therapeutic Radiology and Oncology Consensus Panel. Int J Radiat Oncol Biol Phys 1997;37:1035–1041.

8 Kramer SA, Kline WA Jr, Farham R, Carson CC, Cox EB, Hinshaw W, Paulson DF: Prognosis of patients with stage D1 prostatic adenocarcinoma. J Urol 1981;125:817–819.

9 Whittington R, Malkowicz SB, Barnes MM, Broderick GA, van Arsdalen K, Dougherty MJ, Wein AJ: Combined hormonal and radiation therapy for lymph node-positive prostate cancer. Urology 1995;46:213–219.

10 Roach M 3rd, DeSilvio M, Valicenti R, Grignon D, Asbell SO, Lawton C, Thomas CR Jr, Shipley WU: Whole-pelvis, 'mini-pelvis', or prostate-only external beam radiotherapy after neoadjuvant and concurrent hormonal therapy in patients treated in the Radiation Therapy Oncology Group 9413 trial. Int J Radiat Oncol Biol Phys 2006;66:647–653.

Dr. Gregor Goldner
Department of Radiotherapy and Radiobiology, University Hospital of Vienna
Währinger Gürtel 18–20, AT–1090 Vienna (Austria)
Tel. +43 1 40400 2692, Fax +43 1 40400 2693, E-Mail Gregor.Goldner@akhwien.at

Moser L, Schostak M, Miller K, Hinkelbein W (eds): Controversies in the Treatment of
Prostate Cancer. Front Radiat Ther Oncol. Basel, Karger, 2008, vol 41, pp 77–85

Radiotherapy in Biochemical Recurrences after Surgery for Prostate Cancer

Stefan Höcht   Gunnar Lohm   Lutz Moser
Wolfgang Hinkelbein

Department of Radiation Oncology and Radiotherapy, Charité Universitätsmedizin Berlin,
Campus Benjamin Franklin, Berlin, Germany

Abstract

A biochemical recurrence following prostatectomy is often diagnosed in relatively young and healthy men, and hence deemed very relevant concerning life, given the generally high life expectancy of these patients. Therefore, there is a need for a therapy that offers a long-term chance of cure. Following salvage radiotherapy in large multicenter series, about 45% of the patients treated are in biochemical complete remission 4 years after radiotherapy. The best chances of response are in those patients in whom none of the established risk factors, that will be discussed, are present. Given the established curative potential of salvage radiotherapy and the fact that there are no therapeutic alternatives with a realistic chance of cure, the rather moderate rates of side effects seem acceptable.
Copyright © 2008 S. Karger AG, Basel

Radiotherapy (RT) and surgery offer equal chances in the treatment of prostate cancer with respect to local control and cure of the disease. Differences in potential long-term side effects and the longer follow-up times available for the prostatectomy series are the main reasons why surgery is the preferred option for patients with an age of 65 years or less. In patients older than 65 years, the long-term rate of incontinence is steadily rising after surgery, making this option less advantageous and, vice versa, RT more and more the therapy of choice.

Following surgery, the diagnosis of biochemical recurrence is far easier than after RT. Progression is stated after prostatectomy with a median of 2–3 years, whereas it takes approximately 5 years after RT. Therefore, salvage therapies following radical prostatectomies are usually initiated earlier [1]. These 2 facts lead to the situation that biochemical recurrence following prostatectomy is often diagnosed in relatively young and healthy patients and hence deemed much more relevant concerning life than in the typically elderly patients treated with RT, to whom in general an expectant management or palliative hormone therapy will be offered [2, 3]. Men with locally advanced disease, that is >pT2c, are especially prone to a high risk of local progression after surgery. Several prospective randomized studies on postoperative adjuvant irradiation in these patients have been published, demonstrating both the likelihood of local progression as the cause of a biochemical failure in up to 50% of patients as well as the efficiency of adjuvant irradiation [4, 5]. Whether adjuvant irradiation is superior to early salvage RT as soon as there is evidence of biochemical recurrence is still a matter of debate, although, according to the basic principles of radiation oncology, this has to be expected [5, 6].

The decision to treat a biochemical recurrence in prostate cancer with irradiation will always be accompanied by the possibility of a misjudgement of the situation, leading to an unnecessary and, even worse, potentially harmful therapy as the patient may in fact suffer from distant metastasis. To develop means to judge the likelihood of success is therefore a prerequisite for further refinements in the decision-making process.

Whether the pelvic lymphatics should be treated in primary radiation therapy for prostate cancer still is not clear at all, and the first large-scale, and therefore adequately powered, phase III study on that topic that has been fully published has not offered helpful conclusions hereon [7]. Moreover, in the treatment of a biochemical recurrence there seems to be a sort of consensus that recurrences in the pelvic lymphatics should be managed as systemic disease not amenable to local treatment modalities. Therefore, the rate of patients in whom the pelvic lymph nodes are treated during salvage irradiation is generally very low and below 10% in most published series [8–10].

In those patients in whom the pelvic lymphatics are treated by RT, this mainly is in palliative intent due to hormone-insensitive disease causing complaints by obstruction or compression of lymphovascular drainage. Alleviation of the symptoms is often achieved in these patients, but there are only few reports published dealing with that topic; at least in part this may be due to the limited prognosis of this negatively selected patient population. The other article in this section focuses on patients with a suspected isolated local recurrence.

There is no consensus on staging procedures prior to the initiation of salvage RT. Digital rectal examination and, to a lesser extent, transrectal ultrasonography are cost-efficient maneuvers that should always be done, and, in case of a suspicious finding, histologic confirmation of the suspected recurrence should be attempted. Although some authors still recommend a computed tomography of the abdomen and pelvis, due to the very low sensitivity of this examination cross-sectional diagnostics in fact are not very helpful [11], at least as long as the prostate-specific antigen (PSA) values are below 1.0 ng/ml; even more sophisticated diagnostic tools such as choline-positron emission tomography, magnetic resonance imaging and capromab pendetide scintigraphy (ProstaScint) will be of limited help [12–18]. On the other hand, one should keep in mind that postoperatively many parts of the prostatic fossa are not accessible to a transrectal biopsy and that whilst a positive biopsy may facilitate the decision to irradiate, it does not change the management itself [19, 20].

A considerable number of publications on salvage RT for biochemical recurrence in prostate cancer have been published in recent years and some of them report on large series, either as single-center or multicenter reports [8–10, 21–23]. In these studies, a variety of prognostic parameters have been evaluated. The retrospective nature of this knowledge should be kept in mind when it comes to clinical decision-making processes and cautiousness in their application on an individual patient is mandatory.

From a principle point of view, 2 different scenarios should be distinguished. Patients in whom the PSA value never reached an undetectable range postoperatively (persistently detectable PSA, PD-PSA) and patients in whom PSA postoperatively was below the level of detectability and began to rise later. In some PD-PSA patients, the source of the PSA is a lymph node or bony metastasis already present initially, hence, it is not surprising that many reports state a lower chance of response to salvage RT in that situation, although there is no consensus hereon [23–26; for reviews, see 11, 27].

Even more data exist on the impact of the PSA level at the time point when RT starts on the response rates that can be achieved. The higher these values are, the lower the chances of cure seem to be. Recurrences that are palpable or visible by means of ultrasound or magnetic resonance imaging seem to fare worse; whether this still holds true when the level of PSA is taken into account as well is not clear as these parameters obviously are interrelated. Several different cutoff points for PSA values at the time point of starting RT have been reported in the literature. Older publications tend to propose higher values, above 1.5–2.0 ng/ml, while more recent papers suggest values around 1.0 ng/ml. In our opinion, it is not unlikely that the PSA value at RT start is not a discrete but a continuous parameter, making it likely that an early start of salvage RT is an advisable strategy. Unpublished data on 162 patients treated at our institution, the Department of Radiation Oncology of the Charité Campus Benjamin Franklin in Berlin, offer further support to this assumption [fig. 1].

The definition of obvious progression after prostatectomy is of importance herein. In PD-PSA situations different opinions exist, ranging from an isolated rise to multiple consecutive rises. Additionally, in delayed-rise PSA patients a val-

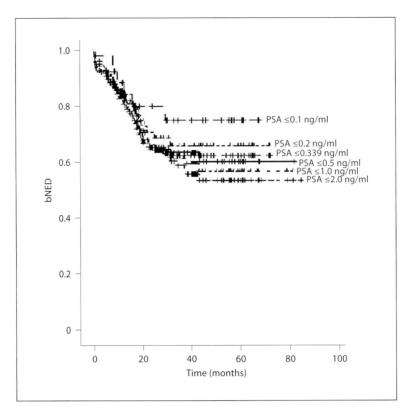

Fig. 1. Biochemical recurrence-free survival (bNED) of 162 patients treated with salvage RT after surgery for prostate cancer at the Department of Radiation Oncology, Charité, Berlin. Outcomes separated with respect to the PSA value at the time salvage RT started.

ue above 0.2 ng/ml has often been deemed necessary for confirmation. Besides uncertainties in the evaluation of PSA kinetics at very low levels, the disappointing precision of PSA testing prior to the introduction of supersensitive test kits may have been a reason for these definitions [3, 28]. The just recently published proposal for a standardized definition of biochemical progression after prostatectomy, suggesting a PSA value of 0.4 ng/ml accompanied by a further rise, is not suitable for salvage RT because it is focusing on distant metastasis as the relevant endpoint [29].

The development of PSA kinetics over time, details from the patient's chart especially concerning details of the operative procedure and pathology report help in defining criteria that make salvage RT more or less likely to be beneficial. Indicators of a poor prognosis are a short interval from surgery to the time the rising of the PSA was detected, a short PSA doubling time or high PSA velocity, a tumor that had without any doubt been resected completely, a Gleason score of 8–10 and an infiltration of the tumor into the seminal vesicles. Even a Gleason score of 7 may be disadvantageous [11, 28]. A PSA doubling time prior to any therapy is a bad sign whatever therapy may be chosen [30].

The largest multicenter study that has been reported on in a full paper is the study by Stephenson et al. [10], documenting the outcome of 501 patients [28]. In that paper there is a flow chart analysis of 356 patients treated without additional hormonal manipulations. Favorable outcomes are shown especially in patients who exhibit only 1 of the poor prognosis indicators mentioned above.

Three-dimensional conformal RT nowadays is the standard not only in salvage RT. Intensity-modulated RT techniques have not yet shown any advantages with respect to clinical or biochemical outcome parameters. Given the existing difficulties in defining the adequate planning target volume in salvage RT, it seems rather unlikely that intensity-modulated RT will be advantageous in general, although in some situations, for instance in patients with a histologically confirmed pararectal nodule, the opposite may be true. There are no large-scale studies on the location of residual or recurrent malignant prostatic tissue after surgery that would guide the decision on which volume should be treated in salvage RT. Many institutions include the prostatic fossa, the bladder neck, the vesicourethral anastomosis and any surgical clips in that area in their standard planning target volumes. The former area of the seminal vesicles or at least their base is often included, but care has to be taken not to include too much rectal volume when doing so.

The standard approach is RT administered with 5 fractions a week of 1.8–2.0 Gy each to a total dose of 64–70 Gy. There is no clear dose-response relationship in salvage RT. Whereas small patient series did suggest a correlation of RT dose and biochemical control, the large-scale multicenter publications with 501 and 911 patients analyzed could not corroborate this finding [10, 22, 23, 31]. To some extent this is quite astonishing, as in primary RT of prostate cancer, dose-response relationships have been described very often [32, 33].

The results of salvage RT are difficult to interpret, not only with respect to the results themselves, but also with respect to the response criteria chosen. Failure definitions after salvage RT are, for instance, a PSA value of >0.4 ng/ml 1 year after salvage RT or any PSA value >0.2 ng/ml following salvage RT, 2 PSA measurements >0.3 ng/ml or 2 PSA rises after achieving a nadir or a rise of more than 0.1 ng/ml above nadir followed by a further increase [8, 10, 21, 22]. These variable criteria definitely do not facilitate interpretation of the situation and make comparisons between the reports very difficult. Generally speaking, in the larger multicenter series, 45% of the patients treated were in biochemical complete remission 4 years after RT and 35% after 5 years [10, 22]. Smaller series do sometimes report more favorable outcomes. The further course of the disease is by now unknown in those patients who exhibit an incomplete response to salvage RT. This phenomenon may sometimes be solely due to inadequate follow-up times. Two thirds of the

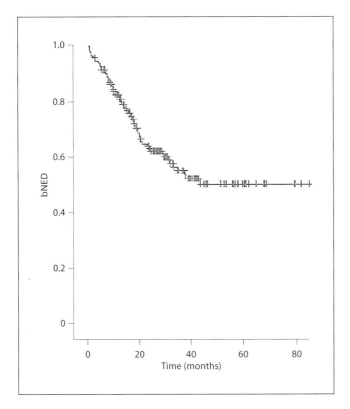

Fig. 2. Biochemical recurrence-free survival (bNED) of 162 patients treated with salvage RT after surgery for prostate cancer at the Department of Radiation Oncology, Charité, Berlin.

patients will achieve the PSA nadir within a year after RT and in some rare cases it may take up to 3 years [8]. On the other hand, it has to be expected that many of the patients with an incomplete response will in the long run suffer from further disease progression.

The best chances of response are found in those patients in whom none of the risk factors mentioned above is present. As the underlying biology of the disease in these men is in itself very favorable, follow-up times of 4–5 years are probably not long enough to evaluate their outcome. Therefore, today there is still some uncertainty about whether salvage RT really does offer a long-term chance of cure. Our own results mentioned earlier do exhibit a stable plateau in the Kaplan-Meier chart at about 50% that is reached after about 4 years (fig. 2). When discussing these data, one should keep in mind that men with a biochemical recurrence of prostate cancer that develops late after surgery and shows a long PSA doubling time do have a quite favorable prognosis even without any therapy [2, 3].

Especially with respect to this fact, acute and chronic side effects of RT are of importance. Although the distorted anatomy after surgery inevitably leads to a relevant portion of the bladder that is included in the treated volume, acute genitourinary (GU) side effects are very moderate and tend to be even lower than in patients under primary RT for prostate cancer [21, 34]. Only 3% grade III GU side effects have to be expected. Severe late GU side effects are rare events. In contrast, Katz et al. [21] reported a high rate of anastomotic strictures that made interventions necessary. However, problems like these are not at all rare events in patients after surgery without adjuvant or salvage RT, making it difficult to attribute them as side effects exclusively caused by RT [35]. Therefore, the actual rate of grade III GU side effects of salvage RT seems to be acceptable.

Mild to moderate proctitis and fecal urge or sometimes incontinence are typical gastrointestinal (GI) side effects during salvage RT. Usually they are of grade I or II and treatment interruptions due to GI toxicity are very rare. The frequency of late GI toxicity, mainly chronic proctitis, is 10–20% for grades I and II and below 5% for grade III [11]. The long-term sequelae on potency are not well documented. Both modalities, surgery and radiation therapy, do have a negative impact on erectile function and the effect of a combination of them is not to be expected to be better than either of the parts.

In conclusion, salvage RT for biochemical recurrence after surgery in prostate cancer is a well-tolerated therapy, offering a chance of cure or at least long-term freedom from progression for 20–40% of the men treated [36]. The impact of additional hormone therapies is still under evaluation.

References

1 Stephenson AJ, Eastham JA: Role of salvage radical prostatectomy for recurrent prostate cancer after radiation therapy. J Clin Oncol 2005;23: 8198–8203.

2 Freedland SJ, Humphreys EB, Mangold LA, Eisenberger M, Dorey FJ, Walsh PC, Partin AW: Risk of prostate cancer-specific mortality following biochemical recurrence after radical prostatectomy. JAMA 2005;294:433–439.

3 Pound CR, Partin AW, Eisenberger MA, Chan DW, Pearson JD, Walsh PC: Natural history of progression after PSA elevation following radical prostatectomy. JAMA 1999;281:1591–1597.

4 Bolla M, van Poppel H, Collette L, van Cangh P, Vekemans K, Da Pozzo L, de Reijke TM, Verbaeys A, Bosset JF, van Velthoven R, Maréchal JM, Scalliet P, Haustermans K, Piérart M, European Organization for Research and Treatment of Cancer: Postoperative radiotherapy after radical prostatectomy: a randomised controlled trial (EORTC trial 22911). Lancet 2005;366:572–578.

5 Höcht S, Hinkelbein W: Postoperative radiotherapy for prostate cancer. Lancet 2005;366:524–525.

6 Coen JJ, Zietman AL, Thakral H, Shipley WU: Radical radiation for localized prostate cancer: local persistence of disease results in a late wave of metastasis. J Clin Oncol 2002;20:3199–3205.

7 Roach M III, DeSilvio M, Lawton C, Uhl V, Machtay M, Seider MJ, Rotman M, Jones C, Asbell SO, Valicenti RK, Han S, Thomas CR Jr, Shipley WS; Radiation Therapy Oncology Group 9413: Phase III trial comparing whole-pelvic versus prostate-only radiotherapy and neoadjuvant versus adjuvant combined androgen suppression: Radiation Therapy Oncology Group 9413. J Clin Oncol 2003;21:1904–1911.

8   Ward JF, Zincke H, Bergstralh EJ, Slezak JM, Blute ML: Prostate specific antigen doubling time subsequent to radical prostatectomy as a prognosticator of outcome following salvage radiotherapy. J Urol 2004;172:2244–2248.

9   Pisansky TM, Kozelsky TF, Myers RP, Hillman DW, Blute ML, Buskirk SJ, Cheville JC, Ferrigni RG, Schild SE: Radiotherapy for isolated serum prostate specific antigen elevation after prostatectomy for prostate cancer. J Urol 2000;163:845–850.

10 Stephenson AJ, Shariat SF, Zelefsky MJ, Kattan MW, Butler EB, Teh BS, Klein EA, Kupelian PA, Roehrborn CG, Pistenmaa DA, Pacholke HD, Liauw SL, Katz MS, Leibel SA, Scardino PT, Slawin KM: Salvage radiotherapy for recurrent prostate cancer after radical prostatectomy. JAMA 2004; 291:1325–1332.

11 Bowers Hayes S, Pollack A: Parameters for treatment decisions for salvage radiation therapy. J Clin Oncol 2005;23:8204–8211.

12 Cher ML, Bianco FJ Jr, Lam JS, Davis LP, Grignon DJ, Sakr WA, Banerjee M, Pontes JE, Wood DP Jr: Limited role of radionuclide bone scintigraphy in patients with prostate specific antigen elevations after radical prostatectomy. J Urol 1998;160: 1387–1391.

13 Seltzer MA, Barbaric Z, Belldegrun A, Naitoh J, Dorey F, Phelps ME, Gambhir SS, Hoh CK: Comparison of helical computerized tomography, positron emission tomography and monoclonal antibody scans for evaluation of lymphnode metastases in patients with prostate specific antigen relapse after treatment for localized prostate cancer. J Urol 1999;162:1322–1328.

14 Kane CJ, Amling CL, Johnstone PA, Pak N, Lance RS, Thrasher JB, Foley JP, Riffenburgh RH, Moul JW: Limited value of bone scintigraphy and computed tomography in assessing biochemical failure after radical prostatectomy. Urology 2003;61: 607–611.

15 Hricak H, Schöder H, Pucar D, Lis E, Eberhardt SC, Onyebuchi CN, Scher HI: Advances in imaging in the postoperative patient with a rising prostate-specific antigen level. Semin Oncol 2003;30:616–634.

16 Wachter S, Tomek S, Kurtaran A, Wachter-Gerstner N, Djavan B, Becherer A, Mitterhauser M, Dobrozemsky G, Li S, Pötter R, Dudczak R, Kletter K: 11C-acetate positron emission tomography imaging and image fusion with computed tomography and magnetic resonance imaging in patients with recurrent prostate cancer. J Clin Oncol 2006;24:2513–2519.

17 Cimitan M, Bortolus R, Morassut S, Canzonieri V, Garbeglio A, Baresic T, Borsatti E, Drigo A, Trovò M: [(18)F] fluorocholine PET/CT imaging for the detection of recurrent prostate cancer at PSA relapse: experience in 100 consecutive patients. Eur J Nucl Med Mol Imaging 2006;33: 1387–1398.

18 Sandblom G, Sörensen J, Lundin N, Häggman M, Malmström PU: Positron emission tomography with C11-acetate for tumor detection and localization in patients with prostate-specific antigen relapse after radical prostatectomy. Urology 2006;67:996–1000.

19 Koppie TM, Grossfeld GD, Nudell DM, Weinberg VK, Carroll PR: Is anastomotic biopsy necessary before radiotherapy after radical prostatectomy? J Urol 2001;166:111–115.

20 Moosbacher MR, Schiff PB, Otoole KM, Benson MC, Olsson CA, Brody RA, Ennis RD: Postprostatectomy salvage radiotherapy for prostate cancer: Impact of pathological and biochemical variables and prostate fossa biopsy. Cancer J 2002;8: 242–246.

21 Katz MS, Zelefsky MJ, Venkatraman ES, Fuks Z, Hummer A, Leibel SA: Predictors of biochemical outcome with salvage conformal radiotherapy after radical prostatectomy for prostate cancer. J Clin Oncol 2003;21:483–489.

22 Pollack A, Hanlon AL, Pisansky TM, et al: A multi-institutional analysis of adjuvant and salvage radiotherapy after radical prostatectomy. Int J Radiat Oncol Biol Phys 2004(suppl)60:186–187.

23 Macdonald OK, Schild SE, Vora SA, Andrews PE, Ferrigni RG, Novicki DE, Swanson SK, Wong WW: Radiotherapy for men with isolated increase in serum prostate specific antigen after radical prostatectomy. J Urol 2003;170:1833–1837.

24 Catton C, Gospodarowicz M, Warde P, Panzarella T, Catton P, McLean M, Milosevic M: Adjuvant and salvage radiation therapy after radical prostatectomy for adenocarcinoma of the prostate. Radiother Oncol 2001;59:51–60.

25 Song DY, Thompson TL, Ramakrishnan V, Harrison R, Bhavsar N, Onaodowan O, DeWeese TL: Salvage radiotherapy for rising or persistent PSA after radical prostatectomy. Urology 2002;60: 281–287.

26 Liauw SL, Webster WS, Pistenmaa DA, Roehrborn CG: Salvage radiotherapy for biochemical failure of radical prostatectomy: a single-institution experience. Urology 2003;61:1204–1210.

27 Bottke D, Wiegel T, Müller M, Höcht S, Altwein JE, Miller K, Hinkelbein W: Strahlentherapie nach radikaler Prostatektomie. Vorgehen bei PSA-Anstieg oder -Persistenz ohne histologische Sicherung eines Lokalrezidivs. Dtsch Arztebl 2004;101:A2255–A2259.

28 Lee AK, D'Amico AV: Utility of prostate-specific antigen kinetics in addition to clinical factors in the selection of patients for salvage local therapy. J Clin Oncol 2005;23:8192–8197.

29 Stephenson AJ, Kattan MW, Eastham JA, Dotan ZA, Bianco FJ Jr, Lilja H, Scardino PT: Defining biochemical recurrence of prostate cancer after radical prostatectomy: a proposal for a standardized definition. J Clin Oncol 2006;24:3973–3978.

30 D'Amico AV, Moul JW, Carroll PR, Sun L, Lubeck D, Chen MH: Surrogate end point for prostate cancer-specific mortality after radical prostatectomy or radiation therapy. J Natl Cancer Inst 2003;95:1376–1383.

31 Anscher MS, Clough R, Dodge R: Radiotherapy for a rising prostate-specific antigen after radical prostatectomy: the first 10 years. Int J Radiat Oncol Biol Phys 2000;48:369–375.

32 Zietman A, DeSilvio ML, Slater JD, Rossi CJ Jr, Miller DW, Adams JA, Shipley WU: Comparison of conventional-dose vs. high-dose conformal radiation therapy in clinically localized adenocarcinoma of the prostate: a randomized controlled trial. JAMA 2005;294:1233–1239.

33 Zelefsky MJ, Fuks Z, Hunt M, Lee HJ, Lombardi D, Ling CC, Reuter VE, Venkatraman ES, Leibel SA: High dose radiation delivered by intensity modulated conformal radiotherapy improves the outcome of localized prostate cancer. J Urol 2001; 166:876–881.

34 Duchesne GM, Dowling C, Frydenberg M, Joseph D, Gogna NK, Neerhut G, Roberts S, Spry N, Turner S, Woo H: Outcome, morbidity, and prognostic factors in post-prostatectomy radiotherapy: an Australian multicenter study. Urology 2003;61:179–183.

35 Begg C, Riedel ER, Bach PB, Kattan MW, Schrag D, Warren JL, Scardino PT: Variations in morbidity after radical prostatectomy. N Engl J Med 2002;346:1138–1144.

36 Stephenson AJ, Pollack A, Scardino PT, Kattan MW: Predicting the outcome of salvage radiotherapy for recurrent prostate cancer after radical prostatectomy. J Clin Oncol 2006;24 (suppl):4514.

Prof. Dr. Stefan Höcht
Klinik für Radioonkologie und Strahlentherapie, Charité Universitätsmedizin Berlin
Campus Benjamin Franklin, Hindenburgdamm 30
DE–12200 Berlin (Germany)
Tel. +49 30 8445 3051, Fax +49 30 8445 2991, E-Mail stefan.hoecht@charite.de

Moser L, Schostak M, Miller K, Hinkelbein W (eds): Controversies in the Treatment of
Prostate Cancer. Front Radiat Ther Oncol. Basel, Karger, 2008, vol 41, pp 86–92

Recurrence following Radiotherapy

F. Desgrandchamps

Department of Urology, Saint Louis Hospital, Paris, France

Abstract

Recurrence after radiotherapy is not uncommon. Facing this situation, physicians have the choice
between numerous possibilities, including simple observation, androgen ablation, salvage radical
prostatectomy, cryotherapy, brachytherapy, high-intensity focused ultrasound, chemotherapy and
nonconventional therapy. There is, however, no standard treatment and each case must be individually discussed.   Copyright © 2008 S. Karger AG, Basel

Recurrence after radiotherapy is not uncommon. A recent update claims that up to
69% of the patients treated for a localized prostate cancer are at risk of recurrence,
with half the recurrences occurring more than 10 years after treatment [1].

Unlike radical prostatectomy, where the diagnosis of recurrence is simply done
by an increasing prostate-specific antigen (PSA), the diagnosis of recurrence after
external beam radiotherapy (EBR) is not simple. The prostate gland is left in situ after radiotherapy and PSA levels decrease only slowly after radiation. PSA nadir levels
are not achieved until at least 18 months after completion of treatment [2].

Defining recurrence after radiation for prostate cancer remains controversial.
A consensus was found 10 years ago. According to this definition, 3 consecutive
PSA increases represent a reasonable definition of biochemical failure after radiation therapy. For clinical trials, the date of failure should be the midpoint between
the postradiation nadir PSA and the first of the 3 consecutive increases. It is likely that this definition will change in the near future as it is difficult to use, delaying
the diagnosis, and as it probably underestimates the real risk of recurrence [3].

The second step in the management of recurrence after EBR is to define whether we face a local or a metastatic disease. For that purpose, digital rectal examination is not of great value and only prostate biopsy gives certitude. Here again, caution is mandatory. Interpreting prostate biopsy after EBR is a difficult exercise,

with a risk of false negatives and also false positives, particularly when biopsies are taken too early; biopsies should not be performed before 18–24 months after completion of the treatment [4].

A general work-up is also needed to rule out distant metastasis: bone scan and computed tomography scan are useful, and among the recent advances in this field, ProstaScint seems to be less helpful than positron emission tomography scan with fluorocholine [5, 6].

PSA doubling time (PSADT) seems to be an accurate test to determine between a local and a metastatic failure, with a cutoff at 6 months. A PSADT of more than 6 months is more consistent with a local failure, a PSADT of less than 6 months indicates a high risk of distant failure, while a high risk of death from prostate cancer is indicated by a PSADT of less than 3 months [7–9].

Once biochemical or local failure is demonstrated after EBR, there is no general agreement among physicians for its management. When asking radiation oncologist or urologists 'What recommendation would you give to a patient demonstrating biochemical or local failure after EBR?', according to the age of the patient, they would answer 'do nothing' in 20–47% of cases, suggest androgen ablation in 37% and propose an active treatment such as salvage prostatectomy or brachytherapy in 3–25% and 12–23% of cases, respectively [10].

Physicians have the choice between numerous possibilities, including simple observation, androgen ablation, salvage radical prostatectomy, cryotherapy, brachytherapy, high-intensity focused ultrasound (HIFU), chemotherapy and nonconventional therapy.

Simple Observation

Biochemical failure is a serious disease. A simple observation shows 5-year clinical disease-free survival rates of 78, 66 and 49% for low-, intermediate- and high-risk cases, respectively, and 10-year clinical disease-free survival rates of 58, 56 and 46%, respectively, in the same groups [11].

Even if in some cases with frail and elderly patients a simple observation is justified, in the vast majority of cases an active option is preferable, considering the poor outcome at 10 years.

Androgen Ablation

Androgen ablation is very popular among physicians facing failure after EBR. However, there is no consensus concerning the criteria used for initiating androgen ablation for PSA failure after EBR. In the survey conducted by Sylvester et al.

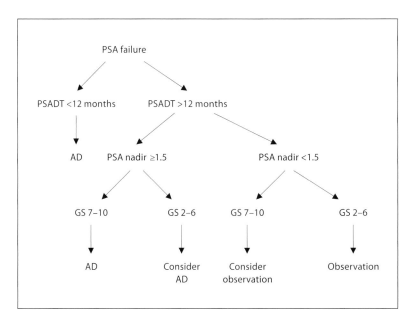

Fig. 1. Proposed algorithm for the management of patients with PSA failure after 3DCRT. AD = Androgen deprivation; GS = Gleason score.

[10], androgen ablation is indicated in the case of clinical failure by 10% of physicians, for an absolute level of PSA by 25% of physicians and for a rate of PSA rise by 65% of them. Again, the cutoff used for PSA varies from one physician to another. ASTRO 3 rise criteria are used by 20% of physicians, PSA above the pretreatment level by 5%, a PSA rise >10 ng/ml by 50%, >20 ng/ml by 20% and >50 ng/ml by 2% [10].

Hormonal manipulation has been compared to simple observation in 248 men with PSA failure (ASTRO) after completing definitive three-dimensional conformal radiotherapy (3DCRT) [12]. Androgen deprivation was started in 59 men, and 89 men who refused were observed. The 5-year freedom from distant metastasis (FDM), cause-specific survival and overall survival rates for the entire group were 76, 92 and 76%, respectively. Gleason score, PSA nadir 1.5 ng/ml, PSADT and the use of androgen deprivation on PSA failure are independent predictors of FDM. Androgen deprivation therapy in patients with PSADT <12 months was associated with a better 5-year FDM rate (57 vs. 78%) and with a longer median time to distant failure (6 vs. 25 months). However, no difference was seen for patients with PSADT >12 months and finally androgen deprivation had no impact on survival [12]. Following these results, an algorithm was proposed for the management of patients with PSA failure after 3DCRT (fig. 1).

Salvage Radical Prostatectomy

Salvage radical prostatectomy has not gained wide acceptance because of the challenges of operating in a radiated field with a significant risk of postoperative complications.

Radiation therapy may interrupt normal wound healing mechanisms. A loss of vessels and fibroblast injury may lead to immature collagen production at the acute phase of wound healing and late radiation effects include atrophy, contraction and fibrosis [13].

Salvage radical prostatectomy is technically difficult, with an increased risk of rectal injury and blood loss. The blood loss is over 1,000 cm^3 in the vast majority of cases, the risk of rectal injury between 0 and 50%. In the postoperative period, the risk of bladder neck contracture is around 20% of cases and the risk of incontinence is far higher than in primary radical prostatectomy (30–80%) [14].

Finally, salvage radical prostatectomy carries a higher risk of positive margins, 60–80% of cases, and is credited with a 5-year biochemical no evidence of disease in 55–69% [14]. Also, the best case for a salvage radical prostatectomy is a patient with a life expectancy of at least 10 years and few comorbidities, a preradiation and preoperative PSA less than 10 ng/ml as well as a preoperative localized clinical stage; however, salvage radical prostatectomy cannot be seen as a standard treatment for failure after EBR.

Salvage Cryotherapy

Globally, salvage cryotherapy leads to 40% biochemical nonevolutive disease at 12–19 months. Complications may occur, including a 10–50% risk of retention and stricture, a 10–80% risk of incontinence, a 20–70% risk of impotence as well as a risk of pelvic pain and rectourethral fistule (up to 11%) [14].

Modern salvage cryotherapy (third generation prostate cryotherapy equipment: argon gas, smaller cryoprobe and brachytherapy-like template) [15] has been evaluated in 1 recent series with adequate follow-up of 4.8 years, giving a 5-year actuarial disease-free survival of 40% (defined as PSA <2 ng/ml above nadir).

Best indications for salvage cryotherapy are older patients with comorbidities, but acceptable operative risk, having a preoperative PSA <10 ng/ml, a Gleason score <8, a clinical stage <T3 and no preoperative hormonal use [14].

Salvage Brachytherapy

Salvage brachytherapy has been performed, but gives a low risk of success, only 34% at 5 years, in old reports [16, 17]. However, there are frequent complications such as the need for additional transurethral resection of the prostate and incontinence. Its applicability is limited after conformational EBR.

Salvage High-Intensity Focused Ultrasound

Salvage HIFU is an attractive option but to date only limited experience exists. A report on 71 patients is available. The main baseline characteristics before HIFU were mean age 67 $\pm$ 5.86 years, mean prostate volume 21.4 $\pm$ 11.1 cm^3 and mean PSA level 7.73 $\pm$ 8.10 ng/ml. All biopsies were positive, with a pre-HIFU Gleason score of 2–6 in 24 patients, 7 in 13 patients and 8–10 in 34 patients. The mean patient follow-up was 14.8 months (range 6–86). After HIFU treatment, 57 (80%) of the 71 patients had negative biopsies, and 43 (61%) of 71 had a nadir PSA level of <0.5 ng/ml. The nadir level was obtained within 3 months. At the last follow-up, 44% of the patients had no evidence of any disease progression. The adverse events related to HIFU included rectourethral fistula in 6%, grade 3 incontinence in 7% and bladder neck stenosis in 17%. No rectal injury occurred [18].

Chemotherapy

Regarding the results obtained with chemotherapy in metastatic hormone-refractory prostate cancer [19], it is likely that chemotherapy will have a place in failure after EBR, but up until now, no data are available to confirm this.

Nonconventional Therapies

Nonconventional therapies are very popular among patients, but only sparse data are available.

Lycopene
Lycopene has been used as dietary supplements in 36 patients with biochemical recurrence (including 24 patients after EBR) and no current hormonal therapy. Mean PSA before lycopene was 4.4 ng/ml (0.8–24.9). Escalating doses (15, 30, 45, 60, 90 and 120 mg/day) were used for 1 year. There was no toxicity, but also no effect on PSA [20].

Vitamin D

A pilot study on the potential role of vitamin D (cholecalciferol) in patients with PSA relapse after definitive therapy has been recently reported [21]. Fifteen patients received 2,000 IU (50 μg) of cholecalciferol daily. In 9 patients, PSA levels decreased or remained unchanged after the commencement of cholecalciferol. This was sustained for as long as 21 months. The median PSADT increased from 14.3 months prior to commencing cholecalciferol to 25 months after commencing cholecalciferol. There were no side effects reported by any patient.

Pomegranate Juice

A phase II study of pomegranate juice for men with rising PSA following surgery or radiation for prostate cancer was recently reported [22]. Pomegranate juice is a major source of antioxidants. Eligible patients had a detectable PSA >0.2 and <5 ng/ml and Gleason score ≤7. Patients were treated with 8 ounces of pomegranate juice daily (Wonderful variety, 570 mg total polyphenol gallic acid equivalents) until disease progression. Mean PSADT significantly increased with treatment from a mean of 15 months at baseline to 54 months after treatment ($p < 0.001$). In vitro assays comparing pre- and posttreatment patient serum on the growth of LNCaP showed a 12% decrease in cell proliferation and a 17% increase in apoptosis ($p = 0.0048$ and 0.0004, respectively), a 23% increase in serum nitric oxide ($p = 0.0085$) and significant ($p < 0.02$) reductions in oxidative state and sensitivity to oxidation of serum lipids after versus before pomegranate juice consumption. There were no serious adverse events reported and the treatment was well tolerated.

Conclusions

Treating a local recurrence after EBR remains an open and difficult question without definitive answer where each case must be individually discussed. This emphasizes the fact that cases for EBR must be selected to reduce the risk of failure.

References

1 Swanson GP, Riggs MW, Earle JD: Long-term follow-up of radiotherapy for prostate cancer. Int J Radiat Oncol Biol Phys 2004;59:406–411.
2 Kuban DA, Thames HD, Shipley WU: Defining recurrence after radiation for prostate cancer. J Urol 2005;173:1871–1878.
3 Consensus statement: guidelines for PSA following radiation therapy. American Society for Therapeutic Radiology and Oncology Consensus Panel. Int J Radiat Oncol Biol Phys 1997;37:1035.
4 Crook JM, Perry GA, Robertson S, Esche BA: Routine prostate biopsies following radiotherapy for prostate cancer: results for 226 patients. Urology 1995;45:624–631.
5 Kahn D, Williams RD, Manyak MJ, Haseman MK, Seldin DW, Libertino JA, Maguire RT: 111Indium-capromab pendetide in the evaluation of patients with residual or recurrent prostate cancer after radical prostatectomy. The ProstaScint Study Group. J Urol 1998;159:2041–2046.

6 Heinisch M, Dirisamer A, Loidl W, Stoiber F, Gruy B, Haim S, Langsteger W: Positron emission tomography/computed tomography with F-18-fluorocholine for restaging of prostate cancer patients: meaningful at PSA <5 ng/ml? Mol Imaging Biol 2006;8:43–48.

7 Amling CL: Biochemical recurrence after localized treatment. Urol Clin North Am 2006;33:147–159.

8 Sartor CI, Strawderman MH, Lin XH, Kish KE, McLaughlin PW, Sandler HM: Rate of PSA rise predicts metastatic versus local recurrence after definitive radiotherapy. Int J Radiat Oncol Biol Phys 1997;38:941–947.

9 D'Amico AV, Moul JW, Carroll PR, Sun L, Lubeck D, Chen MH: Surrogate end point for prostate cancer-specific mortality after radical prostatectomy or radiation therapy. J Natl Cancer Inst. 2003;95:1376–1383.

10 Sylvester J, Grimm P, Blasco J, Meier R, Spiegel J, Heaney C, Cavanagh W: The role of androgen ablation in patients with biochemical or local failure after definitive radiation therapy: a survey of practice patterns of urologists and radiation oncologists in the United States. Urology 2001;58(suppl 1):65–70.

11 Kuban DA, Thames HD, Levy LB, Horwitz EM, Kupelian PA, Martinez AA, Michalski JM, Pisansky TM, Sandler HM, Shipley WU, Zelefsky MJ, Zietman AL: Long-term multi-institutional analysis of stage T1-T2 prostate cancer treated with radiotherapy in the PSA era. Int J Radiat Oncol Biol Phys 2003;57:915–928.

12 Pinover WH, Horwitz EM, Hanlon AL, Uzzo RG, Hanks GE: Validation of a treatment policy for patients with prostate specific antigen failure after three-dimensional conformal prostate radiation therapy. Cancer 2003;97:1127–1133.

13 Tibbs MK: Wound healing following radiation therapy: a review. Radiother Oncol 1997;42:99–106.

14 Touma NJ, Izawa JI, Chin JL: Current status of local salvage therapies following radiation failure for prostate cancer. J Urol 2005;173:373–379.

15 Cresswell J, Asterling S, Chaudhary M, Sheikh N, Greene D: Third-generation cryotherapy for prostate cancer in the UK: a prospective study of the early outcomes in primary and recurrent disease. BJU Int 2006;97:969–974.

16 Grado GL, Collins JM, Kriegshauser JS, Balch CS, Grado MM, Swanson GP, Larson TR, Wilkes MM, Navickis RJ: Salvage brachytherapy for localized prostate cancer after radiotherapy failure. Urology 1999;53:2–10.

17 Beyer DC: Permanent brachytherapy as salvage treatment for recurrent prostate cancer. Urology 1999;54:880–883.

18 Gelet A, Chapelon JY, Poissonnier L, Bouvier R, Rouviere O, Curiel L, Janier M, Vallancien G: Local recurrence of prostate cancer after external beam radiotherapy: early experience of salvage therapy using high-intensity focused ultrasonography. Urology 2004;63:625–629.

19 Tannock IF, de Wit R, Berry WR, Horti J, Pluzanska A, Chi KN, Oudard S, Theodore C, James ND, Turesson I, Rosenthal MA, Eisenberger MA, TAX 327 Investigators: Docetaxel plus prednisone or mitoxantrone plus prednisone for advanced prostate cancer. N Engl J Med 2004;351:1502–1512.

20 Clark PE, Hall MC, Borden LS Jr, Miller AA, Hu JJ, Lee WR, Stindt D, D'Agostino R Jr, Lovato J, Harmon M, Torti FM: Phase I–II prospective dose-escalating trial of lycopene in patients with biochemical relapse of prostate cancer after definitive local therapy. Urology 2006;67:1257–1261.

21 Woo TC, Choo R, Jamieson M, Chander S, Vieth R: Pilot study: potential role of vitamin D (cholecalciferol) in patients with PSA relapse after definitive therapy. Nutr Cancer 2005;51:32–36.

22 Pantuck AJ, Leppert JT, Zomorodian N, Aronson W, Hong J, Barnard RJ, Seeram N, Liker H, Wang H, Elashoff R, Heber D, Aviram M, Ignarro L, Belldegrun A: Phase II study of pomegranate juice for men with rising prostate-specific antigen following surgery or radiation for prostate cancer. Clin Cancer Res 2006;12:4018–4026.

Prof. François Desgrandchamps
Department of Urology, Saint Louis Hospital
1 Avenue Claude Vellefaux
FR–75475 Paris (France)
Tel. +33 1 42 49 96 21, Fax +33 1 42 49 96 16, E-Mail f.dgc@jupiter.chu-stlouis.fr

Moser L, Schostak M, Miller K, Hinkelbein W (eds): Controversies in the Treatment of
Prostate Cancer. Front Radiat Ther Oncol. Basel, Karger, 2008, vol 41, pp 93–102

Secondary Hormonal Manipulation

Axel S. Merseburger[a]   Claus Belka[b]   Klaus Behmenburg[c]
Arnulf Stenzl[a]

Departments of [a]Urology and [b]Radiooncology, Eberhard-Karls University, Tübingen, and
[c]Urology Office, Stuttgart, Germany

Abstract

Patients with advanced prostate cancer under primary androgen deprivation therapy will practically all develop progression, often associated with an asymptomatic increase in prostate-specific antigen. Recent reports are demonstrating an increased use of androgen deprivation therapy as primary or neoadjuvant treatment; however, meager clinical evidence supports the use of such treatment regimens for localized prostate cancer, except in patients with high-risk or locally advanced prostatic disease. Fortunately, the latter tumors might still be prone to some kind of secondary treatment to block androgen receptors in a primary, secondary or tertiary fashion. Secondary hormonal manipulations for affected patients include antiandrogen withdrawal, second-line antiandrogens, direct adrenal androgen inhibitors, estrogens and progestins. We discuss the emerging concept of secondary hormonal manipulation on the basis of the current literature and demonstrate prospective alternative treatment modalities.   Copyright © 2008 S. Karger AG, Basel

Approximately 2–3 years after primary androgen deprivation therapy (PADT), most patients will develop hormone-resistant prostate cancer (HRPC), with rising prostate-specific antigen (PSA) levels as the primary sign of recurrent disease [1]. Among those patients the median survival dramatically decreases to approximately 18 months, with to date no effective treatment with significant improvements of survival [2]. From then, natural progression seems to be unaffectable. Primary hormonal treatment is the common treatment in advanced disease but eventually all patients will unfortunately fail treatment and develop androgen-independent tumors. Fortunately, these tumors might still be prone to some kind of secondary treatment to block androgen receptors (AR) in a primary, secondary or tertiary fashion. In the past several years, there have been new developments and promising research has been performed with secondary hormonal manipulation

(SHM) after the failure of PADT. Nowadays, as nicely presented in the data from the Cancer of the Prostate Strategic Research Endeavor (CaPSURE), luteinizing hormone-releasing hormone agonists represent treatment for 88% of patients who received PADT. Only 3.9% of all patients will receive chemotherapy or additional hormonal therapy as a secondary treatment for prostate cancer [3]. The national trend in the United States, as analyzed by Cooperberg et al. [4], shows a significant increase in the use of PADT throughout all risk groups and treatment modalities. This chapter provides the general evidence for the use of secondary hormonal therapy, focusing on the developments made in the past few years.

Definition of Hormone-Refractory Disease

Unfortunately, all patients on androgen deprivation therapy will fail treatment and develop androgen-independent prostate cancer (AIPC). In the natural progression of prostate cancer towards advanced disease, PADT is followed by some kind of SHM; therefore, it is important to determine a classification. Roughly, there are 3 subgroups: (A) androgen-dependent prostate cancer, (B) AIPC and (C) androgen-independent and hormone-refractory prostate cancer.

Categories B and C would be the eligible groups for a chemotherapy either alone or in combination with SHM therapy in respect to the patient's overall health situation. For the further treatment of the patient, it is important to distinguish between AIPC and HRPC, since patients with AIPC can still benefit from additional hormonal treatment. In HRPC, the benefit of SHM is uncertain.

Rationale for Secondary Hormonal Therapy in Hormone-Sensitive Prostate Cancer

AIPC is defined as measurable progression of prostate cancer despite castrate serum testosterone or progressive disease, as evidenced by at least 1 new lesion on bone scan, growing lymph nodes or increasing serum PSA levels. The latter subgroup of patients is resistant to castration, but to some degree sensitive to SHM [5, 6].

It is known that the AR plays an important role in the course of the disease and studies have shown that amplification of the AR gene is present in advanced HRPC [7, 8]. With disease progression, a mutation of the AR occurs, induced by PADT due to selection. Despite that, several studies have shown at least a 50% decrease in PSA and some degree of clinical benefit in selected patients undergoing SHM due to an individual effect on the AR. Besides, AR can alternatively be activated by factors like growth factors, receptor tyrosine kinases, mitogen-activated protein kinase pathways [9] or activation of AKT (protein kinase B) pathways [10].

Nevertheless, many clinicians fear the side effects and toxicity of these therapies. In this review, we will recommend the treatment options, with special attention to the mostly mild side effects and supplementary medication.

Orchiectomy

Primary castration with subcapsular bilateral orchiectomy was introduced in 1942 and is still considered the gold standard of endocrine treatment of advanced prostate cancer with immediate effect on the plasma testosterone level. There is very little evidence on secondary orchiectomy following initial androgen deprivation therapy and the study by Stone et al. [11] could not describe a benefit [12].

Antiandrogen Withdrawal Therapy

When biochemical progression under PADT occurs, the antiandrogen should be discontinued, since up to 20–30% of patients with PADT will undergo a biochemical response upon withdrawal [13]. The latter phenomenon was initially described by Kelly and Scher [14, 15], while demonstrating a sustained decline in serum PSA levels after discontinuation of the antiandrogen (flutamide). The largest prospective phase III trial showed a >50% decrease in PSA in 13% of patients with objective response in approximately 2% with antiandrogen withdrawal therapy alone [16]. The median duration of the antiandrogen withdrawal response is on average about 5–7 months, in selected cases up to 2 years [17]. Patients who are being treated with androgen deprivation in combination with an antiandrogen at the time of progression can be monitored for the antiandrogen withdrawal syndrome. After antiandrogens have been stopped, further therapeutic interventions to consider include second-line antiandrogens, adrenal androgen inhibition and compounds with estrogenic properties.

Second-Line Antiandrogen Therapy

The effects of antiandrogen therapy, steroidal and nonsteroidal, can be used as second-line therapy by blocking the AR [18]. Bicalutamide, flutamide and nilutamide were evaluated for the ability to induce biochemical or symptomatic responses, hypothetically due to different functional interactions with the AR.

Three studies have shown that in patients treated with higher doses of bicalutamide (150 mg [19, 20] to 200 mg [21]), 20–40% achieved more than 50% reduction in serum PSA after PADT. Bicalutamide is moderately effective in some pa-

Table 1. Toxicities of different antiandrogen therapies

Toxicities	Bicalutamide	Flutamide	Nilutamide
Hot flashes	53	61	22–60
Light adaptation	–	–	12–90
Constipation	22	17	–
Nausea	15	11[1]	10–25
Diarrhea	12	12	–
Anemia	11	6	–
Gynecomastia	9	9	–
Liver abnormalities	7	11	8
Dizziness	–	–	2

Adapted from Daskivich and Oh [18].
[1] Vomiting.

tients with androgen-independent prostate cancer, interestingly in those who received flutamide earlier in their previous medical treatment. When further analyzing the patients included in the Early Prostate Cancer program, who received second-line hormonal therapies (150 mg bicalutamide), approximately 55% of the aforementioned group had a 20% or higher serum PSA decrease after 3 months of second-line antiandrogen treatment [22].

Miyake et al. [23] investigated the efficacy of maximum androgen blockade using flutamide (375 mg daily) as second-line hormonal therapy in 55 patients with advanced hormone-refractory prostate cancer. PSA declines of up to 50% were observed in 22% of included patients. This study revealed a response rate of 6 months with no severe side effects or toxicities.

Concordant responses have been reported for nilutamide following PADT with bicalutamide. Kassouf et al. [24] show PSA response to nilutamide in patients with a previous antiandrogen withdrawal response versus no response of 100 and 18%, respectively. Besides, a previous antiandrogen withdrawal response had a significantly greater chance of responding to nilutamide [24]. This is contrasted by the finding of a study by Nakabayashi et al. [25], where the responders of the cohort of 45 patients did more likely not receive combined androgen blockade. Nilutamide is recommended especially for men who were not initially treated with bicalutamide [26].

To our knowledge, there has been no study so far to evaluate the responses to flutamide following bicalutamide or nilutamide treatment. Ideally, a prospective multicenter study could further investigate this combination. The addition of a second antiandrogen might induce biochemical or symptomatic responses with a survival benefit so far unproven and with moderate toxicity (table 1).

Adrenal Androgen Inhibitors

Up to 10% of androgens are normally secreted by the adrenal glands. An inhibition of testosterone production has been shown to result in symptomatic relief or PSA decline after failure of PADT. For the diagnosed AIPC patient, the following common adrenal androgen inhibitors were available in 2007.

Corticosteroids
Corticosteroids are frequently used in a highly palliative setting to reduce pain in advanced bone-metastasized disease. Studies have shown a reduction of pain in up to 40% of treated men using either prednisone [27], dexamethasone or hydrocortisone [28]. However, the aforementioned study by Tannock et al. [27] also suggests a benefit for quality of life in AIPC when treated with daily doses of 7.5–10 mg. This drug group inhibits secretion of adrenocorticotropic hormone, inducing a negative feedback and eventually decreasing the testosterone production in the adrenal glands. When giving 40 mg/day, Kelly et al. [29] could demonstrate a posttherapy decline in PSA levels after hydrocortisone treatment. Due to the setting of the studies with no randomized controlled trials, there is no evidence-based recommendation for an optimal dosage; hence, there is no doubt that in advanced symptomatic disease corticosteroids play an important role.

Ketoconazole
This inhibitor of cholesterol synthesis is generally used as a temporary antifungal treatment that interferes with cytochrome 3A4 [13], suppresses adrenal testosterone and might even apply direct cytotoxic effects on prostate cancer cells. Investigations on high-dose ketoconazole (400 mg 3 times daily) alone or in combination with hydrocortisone have reported diverging response rates of 50% in 27–62% of patients [16, 30, 31]. Therapy-associated toxicities like nausea, diarrhea, liver failure or skin changes might be reasons to stop this approach; however, promising results from phase II studies could demonstrate similar response rates of 55% with significantly reduced side effects [32]. Recently, a study by Nakabayashi et al. [33] could confirm that low-dose ketoconazole is associated with a PSA response rate comparable to high-dose ketoconazole as secondary hormonal therapy in patients with AIPC. The investigation demonstrated that 39 of 138 eligible patients (28.3%, 95% confidence interval 20.9–36.6%) treated with lower dose experienced PSA declines of $\geq 50\%$. The median time to disease progression or dose escalation on low-dose ketoconazole was 3.2 months (range 0.1–61 months). In summary, low-dose ketoconazole treatment (200 mg 3 times daily) should be given the advantage in second-line therapy.

Aminoglutethimide

These inhibitors of adrenal steroidogenesis initially showed promising results with PSA responses of 30% when combined with a corticosteroid [34]. In combination with steroids, a response of 30% was found, but prospective randomized studies could demonstrate that the response was mainly due to the application of hydrocortisone [35]. However, aside from vague clinical advantage, fatigue, orthostatic hypotension, nausea, skin rash and ataxia are frequent. Therefore, since evidence-based medicine criteria appear to be lacking, at the current time there is no clinical acceptance of the routine use of aminoglutethimide.

Estrogens

Estrogen receptors are overexpressed in advanced prostate cancer tissue, building the rationale for clinical application and investigation of estrogen therapies. The result of the suppression of the pituitary gland's luteinizing hormone-releasing hormone production is achieved within 1–2 weeks. As demonstrated by the investigation of Smith et al. [36], in which diethylstilbestrol (DES) was given at 1 mg/day in 21 patients following antiandrogen withdrawal, 43% of the cohort experienced a PSA decline of more than 50% and the survival at 2 years was 63%. Klotz et al. [37] compared oral DES at either 3 mg daily or 2 mg daily combined with 1 mg warfarin in 32 patients with HRPC. The main problems associated with oral DES therapy were the severe side effects, with one third of the patients developing a deep venous thrombosis and 7% suffering from myocardial infarction or ischemic attacks, so that the application of higher daily oral doses of 1 mg/day was omitted.

Recent developments in transdermal estrogen-based therapies have shown to induce PSA responses of more than 50% with virtually no cardiovascular toxicity compared to traditional estrogens. Ockrim et al. [38] evaluated 20 patients with estradiol patches on hormones, disease progression and toxicity. All patients had a castrate testosterone level within 3 weeks, at a follow-up time of 15 months, 19 of 20 patients were without recurrence [38]. The use of transdermal estrogens preventing first-pass hepatic metabolism, which avoids hepatic enzyme induction effects in substantially reduced cardiovascular risk, might bring a renaissance for estradiol therapy [39–41].

Progestins

Namely 3 progestins, megestrol acetate, medroxyprogesterone acetate and cyproterone acetate, were evaluated and used in the treatment of AIPC. All could demonstrate some degree of PSA responses (8–13%, but no survival benefit), overall health benefit and reduction of pain from metastatic disease in the bone [42–44]. Major side effects include liver toxicity, thrombophlebitis and fluid retention.

AR-Adapted Therapy?

AIPC includes a heterogeneous group of patients with known diverging expression of AR, various mechanisms like secondary signaling pathways and receptor mutations in the cancerous tissue [45, 46].

Chen et al. [47] could show that an increase in AR expression is associated with resistance to antiandrogen therapy. Palmberg et al. [48] found AR gene amplification in 10 of 77 cases (13%). The latter expression was significantly associated with a favorable response to second-line combined androgen blockade. When treating AIPC, it might be of importance to evaluate the individual patient's AR status or even monitor possible changes in progressive disease with, for example, bone marrow examinations [49].

Homeostasis in reproductive tissues requires integration of hormonal and inflammatory signals. Zhu et al. [50] recently discovered that proinflammatory signals switch repressed steroid hormone receptors into transcriptional activators by targeting TAB2, an adaptor protein that tethers corepressors. These findings might have implications for the treatment of endocrine-resistant cancers like advanced prostate cancer [51]. This phenomenon may provide insight into the development of new diagnostic and treatment strategies for advanced prostate cancer.

Conclusion and Future Developments

The goal of this chapter was to review the contemporary value of SHM as a treatment for patients having hormone-independent prostatic disease.

From the data shown above, it is obvious that we do not yet have an ideal method of SHM; therefore, the options and available evidence should be discussed with the patient. Since secondary hormonal therapies are palliative in nature and have not been associated with survival benefit, the choice of treatment should consider the associated toxic side effects. Taken together, up to now, low-dose ketoconazole seems to be the most beneficiary SHM treatment with moderate side effects.

Further substances (calcitriol, follicle-stimulating hormone, mifepristone and liarozole) are under investigation and may bring additional treatment options in the therapy of AIPC. Monoclonal antibodies and so-called small molecule drugs like tyrosine kinase inhibitors or endothelial receptor antagonists open a novel research frontier in the fight against prostate cancer.

References

1 Heidenreich A, Ohlmann CH: Treatment options for hormone-refractory prostate cancer. Urologe A 2005;44:1303.

2 Eisenberger MA, Blumenstein BA, Crawford ED, Miller G, McLeod DG, Loehrer PJ, Wilding G, Sears K, Culkin DJ, Thompson IM Jr, Bueschen AJ, Lowe BA: Bilateral orchiectomy with or without flutamide for metastatic prostate cancer. N Engl J Med 1998;339:1036.

3 Kawakami J, Cowan JE, Elkin EP, Latini DM, DuChane J, Carroll PR; CaPSURE investigators: Androgen-deprivation therapy as primary treatment for localized prostate cancer: data from Cancer of the Prostate Strategic Urologic Research Endeavor (CaPSURE). Cancer 2006;106:1708.

4 Cooperberg MR, Grossfeld GD, Lubeck DP, Carroll PR: National practice patterns and time trends in androgen ablation for localized prostate cancer. J Natl Cancer Inst 2003;95:981.

5 Newling D, Fossa SD, Andersson L, Abrahamsson PA, Aso Y, Eisenberger MA, Khoury S, Kozlowski JS, Kelly K, Scher H, Hartley-Asp B: Assessment of hormone refractory prostate cancer. Urology 1997;49:46.

6 Newling DW: Second-line treatment of metastatic prostatic carcinoma. Urol Res 1997;25(suppl 2): S73.

7 Culig Z, Hobisch A, Bartsch G, Klocker H: Expression and function of androgen receptor in carcinoma of the prostate. Microsc Res Tech 2000;51:447.

8 Debes JD, Tindall DJ: The role of androgens and the androgen receptor in prostate cancer. Cancer Lett 2002;187:1.

9 Klocker H, Culig Z, Eder IE, Nessler-Menardi C, Hobisch A, Putz T, Bartsch G, Peterziel H, Cato AC: Mechanism of androgen receptor activation and possible implications for chemoprevention trials. Eur Urol 1999;35:413.

10 Merseburger AS, Hennenlotter J, Simon P, Muller CC, Kuhs U, Knuchel-Clarke R, Moul JW, Stenzl A, Kuczyk MA: Activation of the PKB/Akt pathway in histological benign prostatic tissue adjacent to the primary malignant lesions. Oncol Rep 2006;16:79.

11 Stone AR, Hargreave TB, Chisholm GD: The diagnosis of oestrogen escape and the role of secondary orchiectomy in prostatic cancer. Br J Urol 1980;52:535.

12 Bishop MC, Lemberger RJ, Selby C, Lawrence WT: Oestrogen dosage in prostatic cancer: the threshold effect? Br J Urol 1989;64:290.

13 Lam JS, Leppert JT, Vemulapalli SN, Shvarts O, Belldegrun AS: Secondary hormonal therapy for advanced prostate cancer. J Urol 2006;175:27.

14 Kelly WK: Endocrine withdrawal syndrome and its relevance to the management of hormone refractory prostate cancer. Eur Urol 1998;34(suppl 3):18.

15 Kelly WK, Scher HI: Prostate specific antigen decline after antiandrogen withdrawal: the flutamide withdrawal syndrome. J Urol 1993;149:607.

16 Small EJ, Halabi S, Dawson NA, Stadler WM, Rini BI, Picus J, Gable P, Torti FM, Kaplan E, Vogelzang NJ: Antiandrogen withdrawal alone or in combination with ketoconazole in androgen-independent prostate cancer patients: a phase III trial (CALGB 9583). J Clin Oncol 2004;22:1025.

17 Small EJ, Carroll PR: Prostate-specific antigen decline after casodex withdrawal: evidence for an antiandrogen withdrawal syndrome. Urology 1994;43:408.

18 Daskivich TJ, Oh WK: Recent progress in hormonal therapy for advanced prostate cancer. Curr Opin Urol 2006;16:173.

19 Joyce R, Fenton MA, Rode P, Constantine M, Gaynes L, Kolvenbag G, DeWolf W, Balk S, Taplin ME, Bubley GJ: High dose bicalutamide for androgen independent prostate cancer: effect of prior hormonal therapy. J Urol 1998;159:149.

20 Kucuk O, Fisher E, Moinpour CM, Coleman D, Hussain MH, Sartor AO, Chatta GS, Lowe BA, Eisenberger MA, Crawford ED: Phase II trial of bicalutamide in patients with advanced prostate cancer in whom conventional hormonal therapy failed: a Southwest Oncology Group study (SWOG 9235). Urology 2001;58:53.

21 Scher HI, Liebertz C, Kelly WK, Mazumdar M, Brett C, Schwartz L, Kolvenbag G, Shapiro L, Schwartz M: Bicalutamide for advanced prostate cancer: the natural versus treated history of disease. J Clin Oncol 1997;15:2928.

22 Wirth M, Iversen P, McLeod D, See W, Morris C, Armstrong J: Response to second-line hormonal therapy following progression on bicalutamide ('Casodex') 150 mg monotherapy. Eur Urol Suppl 2004;3:223.

23 Miyake H, Hara I, Eto H: Clinical outcome of maximum androgen blockade using flutamide as second-line hormonal therapy for hormone-refractory prostate cancer. BJU Int 2005;96:791.

24 Kassouf W, Tanguay S, Aprikian AG: Nilutamide as second line hormone therapy for prostate cancer after androgen ablation fails. J Urol 2003;169:1742.

25 Nakabayashi M, Regan MM, Lifsey D, Kantoff PW, Taplin ME, Sartor O, Oh WK: Efficacy of nilutamide as secondary hormonal therapy in androgen-independent prostate cancer. BJU Int 2005;96:783.

26 Davis NB, Ryan CW, Stadler WM, Vogelzang NJ: A phase II study of nilutamide in men with prostate cancer after the failure of flutamide or bicalutamide therapy. BJU Int 2005;96:787.

27 Tannock I, Gospodarowicz M, Meakin W, Panzarella T, Stewart L, Rider W: Treatment of metastatic prostatic cancer with low-dose prednisone: evaluation of pain and quality of life as pragmatic indices of response. J Clin Oncol 1989;7:590.

28 Tannock IF, Osoba D, Stockler MR, Ernst DS, Neville AJ, Moore MJ, Armitage GR, Wilson JJ, Venner PM, Coppin CM, Murphy KC: Chemotherapy with mitoxantrone plus prednisone or prednisone alone for symptomatic hormone-resistant prostate cancer: a Canadian randomized trial with palliative end points. J Clin Oncol 1996;14:1756.

29 Kelly WK, Curley T, Leibretz C, Dnistrian A, Schwartz M, Scher HI: Prospective evaluation of hydrocortisone and suramin in patients with androgen-independent prostate cancer. J Clin Oncol 1995;13:2208.

30 Millikan R, Baez L, Banerjee T, Wade J, Edwards K, Winn R, Smith TL, Logothetis C: Randomized phase 2 trial of ketoconazole and ketoconazole/doxorubicin in androgen independent prostate cancer. Urol Oncol 2001;6:111.

31 Small EJ, Baron AD, Fippin L, Apodaca D: Ketoconazole retains activity in advanced prostate cancer patients with progression despite flutamide withdrawal. J Urol 1997;157:1204.

32 Harris KA, Weinberg V, Bok RA, Kakefuda M, Small EJ: Low dose ketoconazole with replacement doses of hydrocortisone in patients with progressive androgen independent prostate cancer. J Urol 2002;168:542.

33 Nakabayashi M, Xie W, Regan MM, Jackman DM, Kantoff PW, Oh WK: Response to low-dose ketoconazole and subsequent dose escalation to high-dose ketoconazole in patients with androgen-independent prostate cancer. Cancer 2006;107:975.

34 Plowman PN, Perry LA, Chard T: Androgen suppression by hydrocortisone without aminoglutethimide in orchiectomised men with prostatic cancer. Br J Urol 1987;59:255.

35 Sartor O, Cooper M, Weinberger M, Headlee D, Thibault A, Tompkins A, Steinberg S, Figg WD, Linehan WM, Myers CE: Surprising activity of flutamide withdrawal, when combined with aminoglutethimide, in treatment of 'hormone-refractory' prostate cancer. J Natl Cancer Inst 1994;86:222.

36 Smith DC, Redman BG, Flaherty LE, Li L, Strawderman M, Pienta KJ: A phase II trial of oral diethylstilbesterol as a second-line hormonal agent in advanced prostate cancer. Urology 1998;52:257.

37 Klotz L, McNeill I, Fleshner N: A phase 1–2 trial of diethylstilbestrol plus low dose warfarin in advanced prostate carcinoma. J Urol 1999;161:169.

38 Ockrim JL, Lalani EN, Laniado ME, Carter SS, Abel PD: Transdermal estradiol therapy for advanced prostate cancer – forward to the past? J Urol 2003;169:1735.

39 Ockrim JL, Lalani el-N, Kakkar AK, Abel PD: Transdermal estradiol therapy for prostate cancer reduces thrombophilic activation and protects against thromboembolism. J Urol 2005;174:527.

40 Ockrim JL, Lalani el-N, Aslam M, Standfield N, Abel PD: Changes in vascular flow after transdermal oestradiol therapy for prostate cancer: a mechanism for cardiovascular toxicity and benefit? BJU Int 2006;97:498.

41 Ockrim J, Lalani el-N, Abel P: Therapy Insight: parenteral estrogen treatment for prostate cancer – a new dawn for an old therapy. Nat Clin Pract Oncol 2006;3:552.

42 Dawson NA, Conaway M, Halabi S, Winer EP, Small EJ, Lake D, Vogelzang NJ: A randomized study comparing standard versus moderately high dose megestrol acetate for patients with advanced prostate carcinoma: cancer and leukemia group B study 9181. Cancer 2000;88:825.

43 de Voogt HJ: The position of cyproterone acetate (CPA), a steroidal anti-androgen, in the treatment of prostate cancer. Prostate Suppl 1992;4:91.

44 Torri V, Floriani I: Cyproterone acetate in the therapy of prostate carcinoma. Arch Ital Urol Androl 2005;77:157.

45 Zhou J, Scholes J, Hsieh JT: Signal transduction targets in androgen-independent prostate cancer. Cancer Metastasis Rev 2001;20:351.

46 Small EJ, Ryan CJ: The case for secondary hormonal therapies in the chemotherapy age. J Urol 2006;176:S66.

47 Chen CD, Welsbie DS, Tran C, Baek SH, Chen R, Vessella R, Rosenfeld MG, Sawyers CL: Molecular determinants of resistance to antiandrogen therapy. Nat Med 2004;10:33.

48 Palmberg C, Koivisto P, Kakkola L, Tammela TL, Kallioniemi OP, Visakorpi T: Androgen receptor gene amplification at primary progression predicts response to combined androgen blockade as second line therapy for advanced prostate cancer. J Urol 2000;164:1992.

49 Cronauer MV, Schulz WA, Burchardt T, Anastasiadis AG, de la Taille A, Ackermann R, Burchardt M: The androgen receptor in hormone-refractory prostate cancer: relevance of different mechanisms of androgen receptor signaling. Int J Oncol 2003;23:1095.

50 Zhu P, Baek SH, Bourk EM, Ohgi KA, Garcia-Bassets I, Sanjo H, Akira S, Kotol PF, Glass CK, Rosenfeld MG, Rose DW: Macrophage/cancer cell interactions mediate hormone resistance by a nuclear receptor derepression pathway. Cell 2006;124:615.

51 Brosens JJ, Lam EW, Parker MG: Inflammation and sex steroid receptors: a motif for change. Cell 2006;124:466.

Prof. Dr. Arnulf Stenzl
Department of Urology, Eberhard Karls University
Hoppe-Seyler-Strasse 3
DE–72076 Tübingen (Germany)
Tel. +49 7071 29 85092, Fax +49 7071 29 5092, E-Mail urologie@med.uni-tuebingen.de

Moser L, Schostak M, Miller K, Hinkelbein W (eds): Controversies in the Treatment of
Prostate Cancer. Front Radiat Ther Oncol. Basel, Karger, 2008, vol 41, pp 103–107

Chemotherapy in Hormone-Refractory Prostate Cancer

Johannes Maria Wolff

Department of Urology, Caritas-Krankenhaus, Bad Mergentheim, Germany

Abstract

Research in the past 3 decades has resulted in new approaches to treat patients with hormone-refractory prostate cancer. Employing the new treatment options, we are now able to prolong survival in these patients. At present, docetaxel given on a 3-week schedule is the standard of care for
patients with hormone-refractory prostate cancer. Several new treatments are under investigation
in phase III trials and will further improve the treatment options for these patients within the next
years.   Copyright © 2008 S. Karger AG, Basel

A lot of research has been conducted on hormone-refractory prostate cancer
(HRPC) and its treatment during the last decades. However, it is only recently that
a chemotherapy regimen that significantly prolongs the survival of patients with
HRPC has been developed. These and other findings have changed the management of HRPC patients and it is likely that ongoing research will yield further improvements.

Prostate-Specific Antigen Progression under Androgen Blockade

Treatment options for patients with rising prostate-specific antigen (PSA) levels
under androgen suppression are various [1]. These patients may still have an androgen-dependent prostate cancer and modifying their current therapy may lead
to a further remission, with a median duration of about 6 months [1]. The addition
of an antiandrogen to a luteinizing hormone-releasing hormone analog as well as

the withdrawal of the antiandrogen in patients undergoing complete androgen blockade results in a PSA reduction in up to 60% of these patients. Furthermore, secondary hormone manipulations such as ketoconazole or estrogens again will result in a PSA response in about two-thirds of patients, with a median duration of about 6 months. Depending on the presence of bone metastases, these patients may have a favorable prognosis [2].

Hormone-Refractory Prostate Cancer

Patients with increasing PSA levels despite further hormone manipulations are at risk of developing HRPC. According to the current guidelines of the European Association of Urology (EAU), these patients must meet the following criteria to be considered as having HRPC: (1) clinical and or radiological progression, (2) 3 consecutive PSA rises 2 weeks apart with an increase of 50% over the nadir and (3) PSA progression despite secondary hormone manipulations with maintained castrate levels of testosterone. Depending on the characteristics at presentation, these patients with HRPC may have a median survival of 4–20 months [1].

It is unclear whether androgen suppression should be maintained in these patients and the androgen suppression status of the patients is only rarely reported in trials [3]. Only few studies have addressed that question. However, it was found that continuous androgen blockade was beneficial in patients with HRPC [4]. Therefore, the current EAU guidelines recommend the continued androgen suppression status in patients with HRPC. However, 2 retrospective studies reported different results: continued androgen suppression resulted in a survival benefit in an ECOG study [3], whereas in a SWOG study it did not [5]. Yet, being retrospective studies, these results should be interpreted with caution.

Chemotherapy in HRPC

The results of 2 pivotal studies suggest that docetaxel-based chemotherapy is the treatment of choice for patients with HRPC. In a large randomized 3-arm study (TAX 327), 1,006 patients with HRPC were selected to receive either mitoxantrone every 3 weeks, docetaxel every 3 weeks or docetaxel weekly [6]. The median age was 68 years with more than 200 patients being older than 75 years. The vast majority had bone metastases, about 200 patients had soft tissue metastases and half the patients had pain at baseline. The median survival of patients who received docetaxel 3-weekly was 18.9 months, which was significantly longer than in those receiving mitoxantrone (16.5 months; p = 0.009). Patients receiving docetaxel

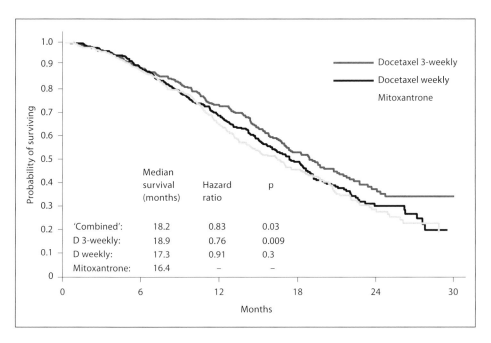

Fig. 1. TAX 327: overall survival of patients with metastatic HRPC treated either with docetaxel (D) 3 weekly, docetaxel weekly or mitoxantrone. Modified from Tannock et al. [6].

weekly had a median survival of 17.4 months (p = 0.36; fig. 1). Furthermore, patients who received docetaxel on either schedule had improved pain control and quality of life in comparison to those who received mitoxantrone. The major adverse events were grade 3/4 neutropenia, diarrhea and neuropathy, being higher in the docetaxel-treated patients.

In the SWOG 9916 study, 674 patients with HRPC were randomized to receive either docetaxel plus estramustine or mitoxantrone and prednisone [7]. At entry, patients were required to have measurable disease. The median age of the patients was 70 years. Median PSA at entry was 84 ng/ml in the docetaxel-treated patients and 90 ng/ml in the mitoxantrone-treated patients. More than 500 patients had bone metastases and over 200 patients had severe pain. Patients treated with docetaxel/estramustine had a significantly greater median survival than those who received mitoxantrone/prednisone (17.7 vs. 15.6 months; p = 0.02; fig. 2). Patients in both groups reported pain relief. Major side effects included neutropenia, nausea, vomiting and cardiovascular events. However, the incidence of adverse events was higher in the docetaxel/estramustine-treated patients.

Median survival of patients treated either with docetaxel alone or docetaxel/estramustine was comparable. As estramustine is associated with an increased risk of side effects, docetaxel plus prednisone is considered to be the standard of care

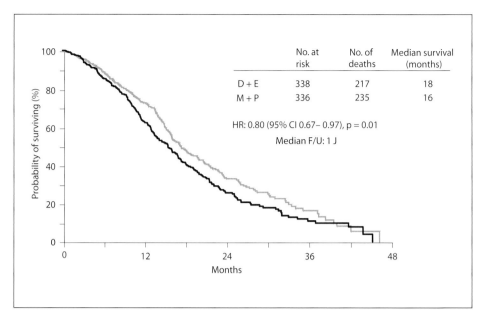

Fig. 2. SWOG 9916: overall survival of patients with metastatic HRPC treated either with docetaxel (D) plus estramustine (E) or mitoxantrone (M) plus prednisone (P). HR = Hazard ratio; CI = confidence interval; F/U = follow-up. Modified from Petrylak et al. [7].

for patients with HRPC. Due to the toxicity profile of the docetaxel regimen, novel combinations and schedules of administration are under investigation. An intermittent regimen was recently evaluated in a multicentre study by the German Uro-Oncology Group (AUO AP33/02) [8]. It was found that intermittent administration of docetaxel/estramustine was as effective as continuous administration. At present, this approach is under investigation in a phase III study by the AUO (AP40/04).

Novel Therapeutic Approaches in HRPC

Research is being carried out on several novel agents for the treatment of HRPC. Recently, the oral platinum analog satraplatin has been evaluated in a phase III study. Three hundred and eighty patients were randomized to receive either satraplatin and prednisone or prednisone alone. However, only 50 patients were enrolled as the study was discontinued by the sponsor. The European Organisation for the Research and Treatment of Cancer (EORTC) followed all patients. Patients receiving satraplatin had a significantly greater median progression-free survival than those receiving prednisone alone (5.2 vs. 2.5 months; p = 0.023). Furthermore, overall survival was improved in the satraplatin-treated patients; however, the difference was statistically not significant (14.9 vs. 11.9 months; p = 0.579). Only minimal adverse events were reported in both treatment groups. Due to these results, satraplatin is under investigation in a large phase III trial as a second-line regimen for patients with HRPC who progressed under first-line cytotoxic chemotherapy.

At present, other novel therapies are under investigation, such as the combination of docetaxel with the vitamin D receptor agonist calcitriol, the endothelin A receptor antagonist atrasantan and the epidermal growth factor inhibitor bevacizumab. The results of these studies are eagerly awaited and new treatment options will hopefully be available for patients with HRPC within the next few years.

References

1 Aus G, Abbou CC, Bolla M, Heidenreich A, Schmid HP, van Poppel H, Wolff J, Zattoni F, European Association of Urology: EAU guidelines on prostate cancer. Eur Urol 2005;48:546–551.

2 Oefelein MG, Agarwal PK, Resnick Ml: Survival of patients with hormone refractory prostate cancer in the prostate specific antigen era. J Urol 2004;171:1525–1528.

3 Taylor CD, Elson P, Trump Dl: Importance of continued testicular suppression in hormone-refractory prostate cancer. J Clin Oncol 1993;11:2167–2172.

4 Manni A, Bartholomew M, Caplan R, et al: Androgen priming and chemotherapy in advanced prostate cancer: evaluation of determinants of clinical outcome. J Clin Oncol 1988;6:1456–1466.

5 Hussain M, Wolf M, Marshall E, Crawford ED, Eisenberger M: Effects of continued androgen-deprivation therapy and other prognostic factors on response and survival in phase II chemotherapie trials for hormone-refractory prostate cancer: a Southwest Oncology Group report. J Clin Oncol 1994;12:1868–1875.

6 Tannock IF, de Wit R, Berry WR, Horti J, Pluzanska A, Chi KN, Oudard S, Théodore C, James ND, Turesson I, Rosenthal MA, Eisenberger MA, TAX 327 Investigators: Docetaxel plus prednisone or mitoxantrone plus prednisone for advanced prostate cancer. N Engl J Med 2004;351:1502–1512.

7 Petrylak DP, Tangen CM, Hussain MHA, et al: Docetaxel and estramustine compared with mitoxantrone and prednisone for advanced refractory prostate cancer. N Engl J Med 2004;351:1513–1520.

8 Miller K, Wülfing C, Lehmann J, et al: Weekly docetaxel plus estramustine for hormone-refractory prostate cancer (HRPC) with intermittent repetition: preliminary results of a multicenter phase II study (AUO AP33/02). J Clin Oncol 2005;23(suppl):4613.

9 Armstrong AJ, Carducci MA: New drugs in prostate cancer. Curr Opin Urol 2006;16:138–145.

10 Sternberg CN, Whelan P, Hetherington J, Paluchowska B, Slee PH, Vekemans K, Van Erps P, Theodore C, Koriakine O, Oliver T, Lebwohl D, Debois M, Zurlo A, Collette L, Genitourinary Tract Group of the EORTC: Phase III trial of satraplatin, an oral platinum plus prednisone vs. prednisone alone in patients with hormone-refractory prostate cancer. Oncology 2005;68:2–9.

Prof. Dr. Johannes Maria Wolff
Department of Urology, Caritas-Krankenhaus
Uhlandstrasse 7
DE–97980 Bad Mergentheim (Germany)
Tel. +49 7931 582 701, Fax +49 7931 582 790, E-Mail johannes.wolff@ckbm.de

Moser L, Schostak M, Miller K, Hinkelbein W (eds): Controversies in the Treatment of
Prostate Cancer. Front Radiat Ther Oncol. Basel, Karger, 2008, vol 41, pp 108–116

A Randomized Phase II Trial Comparing Weekly Taxotere plus Prednisolone versus Prednisolone Alone in Androgen-Independent Prostate Cancer

Sophie D. Fosså

Department of Clinical Cancer Research, Rikshospitalet – Radiumhospitalet Medical Center
and University of Oslo, Oslo, Norway

Abstract

Prednisolone monotherapy has been the standard systemic treatment in many patients with androgen-independent prostate cancer and should today be compared to treatment with Taxotere plus
prednisolone. One hundred and thirty four patients were entered into a randomized phase II study
[arm A: Taxotere plus prednisolone (30 mg/m^2 weekly during 5 of 6 weeks + prednisolone 5 mg orally twice daily); arm B: prednisolone (5 mg orally twice daily)]. Biochemical response at 6 weeks was
the primary outcome parameter, with progression-free and overall survival as secondary outcomes.
Biochemical response at 6 weeks was recorded in 29 of 54 evaluable patients in arm A [54%; 95%
confidence interval (CI) 40–67%] and 13 of 50 patients in arm B (26%; 95% CI 14–38%), with a similar
difference in response rates at 12 weeks. Median progression-free survival was 11 months in arm A
(95% CI 5.8–16.2)and 4 months in arm B (95% CI 2.4–5.6). Median overall survival was 27 months in arm
A (95% CI 19.8–34.1) and 18 months in arm B (95% CI 15.2–20.8). Assessment of pain and quality of life
showed superiority of arm A treatment, without unacceptable toxicity. Taxotere plus prednisolone is
recommended as systemic standard treatment in androgen-independent prostate cancer.

Until 2004, no treatment was available which prolonged survival in patients with
androgen-independent prostate cancer (AIPC) [1]. In the balance between efficacy, side effects, feasibility and expense, small doses of oral prednisolone daily have
for many years represented the standard medical treatment of patients with AIPC
in the Nordic countries [2]. After the reports of promising response rates of

docetaxel (Taxotere; Sanofi-Aventis) in AIPC [3, 4], Norwegian and Swedish clinicians agreed to perform a randomized phase II trial in AIPC patients, comparing weekly Taxotere plus prednisolone (arm A) with prednisolone alone (arm B) to assess treatment efficacy and feasibility.

After publication of the 2 pivotal trials [5, 6] showing life prolongation in AIPC patients receiving Taxotere, the trial was prematurely closed due to a decreasing inclusion rate. In this report, the main findings of the multicenter trial are summarized with reference to the original publication from 2007 [7].

Patients and Methods

Patients
Eligible patients fulfilled the following criteria: (1) histologically proven progressing prostate adenocarcinoma with distant metastases, (2) prostate-specific antigen (PSA) increase in at least 2 blood samples and PSA at trial entry >10 µg/l, (3) serum testosterone within the institution's castration range, (4) no prior chemotherapy or new hormonal agents after the diagnosis of AIPC, (5) ECOG performance status ≤2, (6) age <85 years, (7) no other malignancy during the previous 5 years, except for basocellular skin cancer and (8) sufficient bone marrow function as judged by peripheral blood cell counts.

Treatment
Treatment in arm A consisted of 6 cycles with Taxotere plus prednisolone, each cycle lasting for 6 weeks. Taxotere 30 mg/m^2 was applied on days 1, 8, 15, 22 and 29 as a 1-hour intravenous infusion. Prednisolone 5 mg was given orally twice daily. Patients also used a single oral dose of 32 mg methylprednisolone on the evening before a Taxotere infusion, repeating this medication twice on the 2 following days and once during the third morning. Patients in treatment arm B had prednisolone 5 mg orally twice daily. From week 36 (after 6 cycles), nonprogressing patients from both arms with acceptable drug tolerance continued with prednisolone 5 mg orally twice daily.

The end of treatment was reached in case of progression (see below) or the patient's withdrawal of consent. Subsequent therapy was at the discretion of the clinical investigator, discouraging the use of taxanes.

Toxicity and Dose Modification
The trial protocol contained rules for treatment modifications based on hematological and nonhematological toxicity, but did not consider hyperlacrimation or nail discoloring.

Response Evaluation and Endpoints
The primary endpoint, biochemical response, was initially defined as PSA decrease by ≥50% of the baseline level after the 6-week treatment [8]. After having observed the surge phenomenon during cycle 1 in arm A, it was recommended to continue treatment for at least 12 weeks in spite of transient PSA increase.

Subjective progression was defined as an increase in the performance status/pain/analgesics score [9] by ≥4 points compared to its baseline score.

Progression was defined as biochemical progression, subjective progression or the combination of both, or death, whichever occurred first. Progression-free survival and overall survival were secondary endpoints together with the assessment of safety and quality of life.

Follow-Up
During the first 36 weeks, all patients within the trial received a clinical and hematological examination every sixth week. Thereafter, follow-up visits were scheduled with 3-month intervals in patients remaining in the trial.

Quality of Life
The patients completed the EORTC QLQ-C30 questionnaire [10] before the start of treatment and thereafter every sixth week until they went off the trial.

Data Management and Statistics
Ninety-one patients in each arm were required to prove a 40% response rate in arm A and a 20% response rate in arm B (α: 0.05; β: 0.20). Progression-free and overall survival were assessed by Kaplan-Meier plots.

The scorings of the EORTC QLQ-C30 were transformed following published guidelines [10]. Analyses were restricted to changes at 12 weeks of global quality of life, physical function, pain, fatigue and nausea/vomiting. Clinically significant changes required changes of ≥ 10 points [11].

Results

Patients
Of the 134 randomized patients, 104 and 97 were evaluable at 6 and 12 weeks, respectively (table 1).

Exposure to Treatment
Twenty-four of the 57 eligible patients of arm A had all 6 cycles. Among arm B patients, prednisolone was stopped after 6, 12 and 24 weeks, as the responsible physician opted for alternative treatment in patients with stable disease. A fourth patient from arm B withdrew his consent after cycle 1. After 36 weeks, 14 eligible nonprogressing patients remained in arm B.

Efficacy
Both at 6 and 12 weeks, significantly more patients in arm A than arm B responded biochemically (table 2). At both assessments, fewer patients from arm A than arm B displayed biochemical progression. At 12 weeks, subjective progression was recorded in 6 of 42 patients on arm B (14%) and in 4 of 52 patients on arm B (8%).

In a subanalysis, 12-week changes of serum total alkaline phosphatase (t-ALP) were studied in 72 patients as a possible additional biomarker of efficacy: in pa-

Table 1. Patient characteristics at baseline

a Demographics and biochemical parameters

	Tax + P	P
Randomized	71	63
Eligible[1]	57	52
Evaluable for response[2]		
6 weeks	54	50
12 weeks	52	45
Median age, years	70 (52–81)	72 (54–84)
Median time from diagnosis to		
randomization, months	53 (8–155)	52 (10–231)
Analgesic use		
None	29	28
Nonopioids	19	18
Opioids	9	6
Distant metastases		
Soft tissue only	5	4
Bone metastases+	49	47
Unknown	3	1
Previous radiotherapy		
Yes	21	17
No	36	35
Median baseline PSA	130 (14–1681)	163 (14–2551)
Hemoglobin	13.2 (9.6–15.4)	12.8 (9.9–15.2)
ALP	161 (14–2820)	144 (37–1587)
LDH	245 (121–1740)	224 (158–657)

Figures in parentheses are ranges. Tax = Taxotere; P = prednisolone; ALP = alkaline phosphatase; LDH = lactate dehydrogenase.

[1] Reasons for ineligibility in arm A/B: prior systemic treatment after AIPC diagnosis: 5/3; no progression: 2/2; PSA <10 µg/l: 2/0; incompatible blood tests: 4/6; other cancer: 1/0; other medical condition: 1/0.

[2] Reasons for not being evaluable are given in the text.

b Quality of life scores (EORTC QLQ-C30) in 108 eligible patients with baseline quality of life questionnaire

	Arm A: Tax + P (n = 56)	Arm B: P (n = 52)
Physical function	75 (18.2)	75 (23.6)
Pain	34 (29.1)	29 (29.9)
Fatigue	38 (24.1)	33 (21.3)
Nausea/Vomiting	9 (19.3)	5 (11.7)
Global quality of life	64 (20.9)	65 (22.2)

Data are presented as means with standard deviations in parentheses. Tax = Taxotere; P = prednisolone.

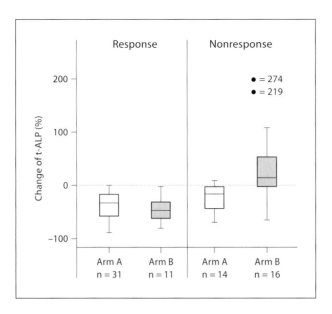

Fig. 1. Change from baseline of t-ALP at 12 weeks and PSA response. Dotted line = baseline; solid line = median; n = number of patients with known t-ALP values. ● = Outliers.

Table 2. Biochemical response (PSA) and physician-assessed clinical improvement by ≥1 point/subjective progression during the first 12 weeks or prior end of study

	Arm A: Tax + P	Arm B: P
6 weeks		
Response	29/54 (54)[1]	13/50 (26)[1]
Stable[2]	22 (41)	24 (48)
Progression	3 (6)	13 (26)
12 weeks		
Response	36/52 (69)[1]	16/45 (36)[1]
Stable[2]	10 (19)	16 (36)
Progression	6 (12)	13 (29)

Figures in parentheses are percentages. Tax = Taxotere; P = prednisolone.
[1] Number of responding/evaluable patients.
[2] Not fulfilling the criteria of response or progression [15].

tients with biochemical response, a ≥50% reduction of t-ALP was noted in 10 of 31 patients from arm A as opposed to 1 of 14 patients in arm B (p = 0.07). Even among nonresponders, more patients from arm A (5 of 11) experienced t-ALP reductions of ≥50% than from arm B (1 of 16; fig. 1). This difference was mainly

Fosså

Table 3. Quality of life evaluation at 12 weeks

	Arm A: Tax + P (n = 48)			Arm B: P (n = 38)		
	improved	unchanged	worse	improved	unchanged	worse
Physical function*	13 (27)	20 (42)	15 (31)	1 (3)	28 (74)	9 (24)
Pain*	25 (52)	16 (33)	7 (15)	6 (16)	19 (50)	13 (34)
Fatigue	18 (38)	13 (27)	17 (35)	11 (29)	10 (26)	17 (45)
Nausea/vomiting	8 (17)	36 (70)	4 (8)	3 (8)	31 (82)	4 (10)
Global quality of life	13 (27)	19 (40)	16 (33)	6 (16)	22 (58)	10 (26)

Data are restricted to patients assessable for quality of life at baseline and at 12 weeks. Figures in parentheses are percentages. * $p < 0.05$.

due to the different t-ALP kinetics in patients with stable PSA: at the 12-week assessment, t-ALP had decreased by $\geq 50\%$ in 4 of 9 patients with stable PSA from arm A, but only in 1 of 12 similar patients from arm B.

Safety and Tolerability

Neutropenia of grade ≥ 3 without neutropenic fever was observed in 2 arm A patients, and no cases of grade ≥ 3 thrombocytopenia were observed. Only 2 patients on arm A had dose reductions.

In arm A patients, nail changes [discoloration, oncholysis (27 patients)], alopecia (9 patients), conjunctivitis/tearing (8 patients) and fatigue (6 patients) were the most frequent nonhematological adverse events (all scored as $\geq$ grade 2). Grade 2 nausea/vomiting was reported in 5 patients from arm A. The only nonhematological toxicity among arm B patients was weight increase >5 kg in 2 patients.

Quality of Life

At 12 weeks, 25 of 48 patients (52%) from arm A and 6 of 38 men (16%) from arm B reported clinically significant pain reduction (p = 0.02; table 3). Further, significantly more patients on arm A recorded improved physical function than on arm B (p = 0.02).

Survival

The median progression-free survival in arm A was 11 months [95% confidence interval (CI) 6–16] and 4 months (95% CI 2–6) in arm B (p = 0.08; fig. 2a). By 1 January 2006, 63 men were dead (arm A: 28; arm B: 35). The median overall survival in arm A was 27 months (95% CI 20–34) and 18 months (95% CI 15–21) in arm B (p = 0.015; fig. 2b).

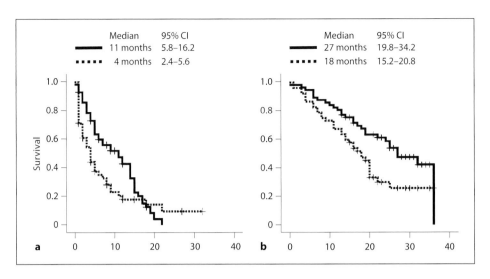

Fig. 2. Taxotere and prednisolone (solid line; 57 patients) versus prednisolone alone (dotted line; 52 patients) in androgen-independent prostate cancer. **a** Progression-free survival. **b** Overall survival.

Discussion

In line with published phase II and phase III trials [3–6], this randomized phase II study demonstrates a 6-week biochemical response rate of 54% in AIPC patients receiving Taxotere, increasing to a PSA response rate of 69% at 12-week assessment, and a median overall survival of 27 months. In patients receiving prednisolone alone, the response rates were 26 and 36%, respectively, and the median overall survival was 18 months. Toxicity was acceptable in both treatment alternatives.

In the present study, patients went off trial in case of clearly defined biochemical progression, observed at any time. However, very early during the trial performance we became aware of a possible 'PSA surge' occasionally observed during the first cycle of arm A.

Similar observations are reported by Fizazi et al. [12] and Fosså et al. [13]. PSA surge might indicate massive cancer kill associated with excessive PSA release. Therefore, we now recommend to delay assessment of biochemical response to the 12-week visit.

The high percentage of pain relief after 12 weeks in arm A was an important clinical finding in line with the results of TAX 327 [5]. When interpreting the positive results of this trial, the much higher cumulative dose of corticosteroids during a 6-week cycle in arm A patients should not be overlooked as a possible contributory factor.

The elevated t-ALP levels in our study are considered mainly to mirror bone alkaline phosphatase. The fact that we observed more pronounced t-ALP decrease in biochemically responding patients from arm A than in those from arm B, with even larger differences in nonresponding patients, made us speculate whether Taxotere has some direct or indirect influence on osteoblast activity. Reduced bone metabolism has been shown to be associated with pain relief and decreased risk for adverse skeletal events in patients with AIPC or other solid tumors, even in the absence of major PSA response, for example during treatment with zoledronic acid [14] or atrasentan [15]. Again, the higher cumulative doses of corticosteroids in arm A should be kept in mind when interpreting the shown t-ALP changes. Associations have been shown between high serum levels of corticosteroids during short periods and reduced osteoblast activity [16].

Albeit based on small numbers in our trial and lack of sufficient statistical power, the 9-month difference in median survival between arm A and arm B was greater than expected from published reports [5, 6], in part possibly explained by the lack of crossover in the present trial.

The low and manageable toxicity in patients on arm A was a positive surprise, particularly the absence of high-grade nausea and vomiting. The 3-week regimen of Taxotere might even be more acceptable in AIPC patients due to less frequent consultations.

Conclusion

The treatment of AIPC patients with Taxotere plus prednisolone leads to biochemical response rates of >50% superior to comparable figures in patients treated with prednisolone monotherapy. Favorable survival and an acceptable toxicity profile further support the future use of Taxotere in these patients. Further investigations are warranted to explore the influence of Taxotere on osteoblast activity.

References

1 Clarke NW, Wylie JP: Chemotherapy in hormone refractory prostate cancer: where do we stand? Eur Urol 2004;46:709–711.
2 Fosså SD, Slee PH, Brausi M, et al: Flutamide versus prednisone in patients with prostate cancer symptomatically progressing after androgen-ablative therapy: a phase III study of the European Organization for Research and Treatment of Cancer Genitourinary Group. J Clin Oncol 2001; 19:62–71.
3 Beer TM, Pierce WC, Lowe BA, Henner WD: Phase II study of weekly docetaxel in symptomatic androgen-independent prostate cancer. Ann Oncol 2001;12;1273–1279.
4 Berry W, Dakhil S, Gregurich MA, Asmar L: Phase II trial of single-agent weekly docetaxel in hormone-refractory, symptomatic, metastatic carcinoma of the prostate. Semin Oncol 2001; 28(suppl 15);8–15.

5 Tannock IF, de Wit R, Berry WR, et al: Docetaxel plus prednisone or mitoxantrone plus prednisone for advanced prostate cancer. N Engl J Med 2004;351:1502–1512.

6 Petrylak DP, Tangen CM, Hussain MHA, et al: Docetaxel and estramustine compared with mitoxantrone and prednisone for advanced refractory prostate cancer. N Engl J Med 2004;351:1513–1520.

7 Fosså SD, Jacobsen AB, Ginman C, et al: Weekly taxotere and prednisolone versus prednisolone alone in androgen-independent prostate cancer: a randomized phase II study. Eur Urol 2007;52:1691–1698.

8 Bubley GJ, Carducci M, Dahut W, et al: Eligibility and response guidelines for phase II clinical trials in androgen-independent prostate cancer: recommendations from the Prostate-Specific Antigen Working Group. J Clin Oncol 1999;17:3461–3467.

9 Hedlund PO, Ala-Opas M, Brekkan E, et al: Parenteral estrogen versus combined androgen deprivation in the treatment of metastatic prostatic cancer. Scand J Urol Nephrol 2002;36:405–413.

10 Aaronson NK, Ahmedzai S, Bergman B, et al: The European Organization for Research and Treatment of Cancer QLQ-C30: a quality of life instrument for use in international clinical trials in oncology. J Natl Cancer Inst 1993;85:365–376.

11 Osoba D, Rodrigues G, Myles J, et al: Interpreting the significance of changes in health-related quality of life scores. J Clin Oncol 1998;16:139–144.

12 Fizazi K, Thuret R, Theodore C, et al: Early PSA rise subsequently followed by PSA decline is a common event in prostate cancer patients responders to chemotherapy. Ann Oncol 2004;15(suppl 3):427.

13 Fosså SD, Vaage S, Letocha H, Iversen J, Risberg T, Johannessen DC, Paus E, Smedsrud T: Liposomal doxorubicin (Caelyx®) in symptomatic androgen-independent prostate cancer (AIPC): delayed response and flare phenomenon should be considered. Scand J Urol Nephrol 2002;36:34–39.

14 Coleman RE, Major P, Lipton A, et al: Predictive value of bone resorption and formation markers in cancer patients with bone metastases receiving the bisphosphonate zoledronic acid. J Clin Oncol 2005;23:4925–4935.

15 Cella D, Petrylak DP, Fishman M, et al: Role of quality of life in men with metastatic hormone-refractory prostate cancer: how does atrasentan influence quality of life? Eur Urol 2006;49:781–789.

16 Klein GL, Bi LX, Sherrard DJ, et al: Evidence supporting a role of glucocorticoids in short-term bone loss in burned children. Osteoporos Int 2004;15:468–474.

Dr. Sophie D. Fosså
Department of Clinical Cancer Research, Rikshospitalet – Radiumhospitalet Medical Center
Montebello
NO–0310 Oslo (Norway)
Tel. +47 2293 4000, Fax +47 2293 4553, E-Mail sdf@radiumhospitalet.no

Moser L, Schostak M, Miller K, Hinkelbein W (eds): Controversies in the Treatment of
Prostate Cancer. Front Radiat Ther Oncol. Basel, Karger, 2008, vol 41, pp 117–125

Hormone-Refractory and Metastatic Prostate Cancer – Palliative Radiotherapy

Lutz Moser   Tina Schubert   Wolfgang Hinkelbein

Charité Universitätsmedizin Berlin, Campus Benjamin Franklin, Berlin, Germany

Abstract

Prostate cancer progression is commonly manifested by obstructive uropathy, regional lymphatic metastases and hematogenous metastases to the axial skeleton. Radiotherapy is a mainstay in the palliation of symptomatic metastatic prostate cancer and is most often used for the palliation of painful metastatic bone lesions, resulting in a relief of pain in about 80–90% of patients and a reduction of analgesics. In metastatic disease compromising the integrity of the spinal cord or a nerve root, radiotherapy can be used as an urgent intervention to minimize neurological dysfunction and local progression or as an adjunct to surgical decompression. Local progression is often associated with hematuria, ureteric obstruction and perineal discomfort. Symptoms of metastatic lymphadenopathy like leg edema and back discomfort caused by pelvic or paraaortic metastases are related to the immediate anatomic structures affected. Radiotherapy for localized hormone-refractory prostate cancer has an excellent local control rate; nevertheless, the prognosis is poor, the majority of patients failing with distant metastasis within few years. The role of radiotherapy in hormone-refractory and metastatic prostate cancer, considering the patient's individual situation, are presented and discussed.

Palliative care improves the quality of life of patients by providing pain and symptom relief, from diagnosis to the end of life (according to WHO). The principal aim is to alleviate the patient's symptoms. For many men, androgen ablation in metastatic prostate cancer is an effective treatment; however, when it fails, the quality of life can quickly degrade. Besides analgesics, different treatment options are available for further palliation in case of local and systemic symptomatic progression. In the following, the opportunities of radiotherapy are demonstrated and discussed.

Symptomatic Skeletal Metastases

The most common site of distant metastases in prostate cancer is the skeleton. The osteoblastic process predominates and gives rise to the typical radiographic appearance often referred to as blastic or sclerotic lesions. In about 50–80% of patients, symptoms from bone metastases manifest as skeletal or neuropathic pain, pathological fractures, hypercalcemia, nerve root damage and spinal cord compression. The goals of treatment are relief of pain, preservation of mobility and function, maintenance of skeletal integrity and preservation of quality of life.

Pain Control, Analgesic Effect

The most common symptom of skeletal metastases is pain, present in the majority of patients with metastatic bone lesions. Typically, the pain is slowly progressive over days to weeks and requires frequently increasing doses of analgesics. Skeletal pain is thought to be induced by a combination of mechanical and biochemical factors resulting in activation of pain receptors in local nerves. Increased blood flow to the metastatic lesions promotes an inflammatory response, with release of cytokines by both the tumor cells and the surrounding tissue.

Besides analgesics and bisphosphonates, localized skeletal pain due to metastatic prostate cancer can be effectively treated with external radiotherapy with an improvement in 50–80% and complete relief in about 20–50% of patients. However, dose and fractionation were not clearly defined for decades. Even in 1992, a consensus meeting on the treatment of bone metastases came to the conclusion that 'the relationships between radiotherapy dose and response duration in terms of pain relief and bone healing are poorly defined and require further investigation' [1]. Thereafter, many retrospective and prospective controlled trials focused on dose and fractionation in symptomatic skeletal metastases.

Fractionation of External Beam Irradiation

Pain relief, in terms of degree and duration, does not depend on the fractionation schedules applied. No significant differences in terms of pain relief and analgesic use were found if single fractions, shorter duration treatments or more protracted regimens were compared in randomized studies [2–10].

The velocity of pain relief was analyzed in one of the randomized studies. Following a single fraction of 8 Gy, the relief of pain was faster, with a reduction of pain in 25 and 50% of patients after 2 and 5 days, respectively. Patients treated with the fractionated regimen noted an initial response after 5 and 10 days, respectively. The maximum relief of pain was reached in both arms after 1 month.

The local palliative efficiency can be expressed as the time to pain progression, rate of pathological fractures and the requirement of local retreatment. Depending on the reported time periods for evaluation and how the results were assessed, the documented duration of pain relief is more than 6 months in at least 50% of patients and the first increase in pain score can be expected after 1 year in 40% of patients [11].

The reported incidence of pathological fractures following palliative radiotherapy of bone metastases is low, varying between 1 and 10%. A suspected higher rate of pathological fractures following a single fraction was only confirmed in 2 of the 9 randomized studies. Despite this difference, the low rates for pathological fractures of 4–5% after a single fraction of 8 Gy should not be the main criteria for treatment decision [9, 10].

Three randomized studies found the rate of re-treatment to be higher following a single fraction than multifractionation regimens [3, 9, 10]. For example, twice as many patients had to be re-treated in the single 8 Gy arm (18%) than following the longer course of 30 Gy in 10 fractions (9%) in the recently published RTOG 97-14 study [3]. Unfortunately, it was not clarified whether there was no medical indication following the more protracted schedule or if there may have been less willingness to give another treatment with respect to more pronounced toxicity from sensitive critical normal structures. A suspected higher acute toxicity associated with that regimen might have led to the decision not to re-treat.

Toxicity
Irrespective of the fractionation schedule chosen, the incidence of grade 2 or greater acute and late toxicity is low, with a rate of approximately 10–15 and 4%, respectively. With regard to acute toxicities, a predominance of gastrointestinal adverse effects like emesis and diarrhea has to be noted. In general, acute toxicity is mild, rarely requiring further supportive care.

Recalcification
There is only 1 report in which the endpoint of skeletal remineralization of osteolytic metastases is studied. Densitometric data obtained by computed tomography before irradiation as well as 6 weeks, 3 months and 6 months thereafter were evaluated. Remineralization was defined as a rise of density in the region of interest of more than 20%. After 6 months, remineralization of the metastatic lesion was found in 58 and 25% of patients of the multifractionation and single-fraction group, respectively (178 vs. 120%, $p < 0.0001$) [3].

Radionuclide Therapy
Metastases to the skeleton are usually multiple; solitary metastases appear in less than 10% of patients. Generalized bone pain due to multiple metastases from carcinomas of the prostate and breast indicates systemic treatment. Radionuclide

therapy with 89-strontium or 153-samarium is effective with an overall bone pain relief in about 60–80% of patients and a median response duration of 2–4 months. Acute side effects contain mild and transient myelosuppression occurring 3–6 weeks after treatment.

Although most published investigations were conducted in patients with several types of tumors, carcinomas of the prostate, breast and bronchi predominated [11]. One controlled randomized study focused on bone pain relief by either external beam irradiation or systemic radionuclide therapy with 89-strontium in patients with hormone-refractory prostate cancer. The efficiency in the treatment groups was found to be the same; however, the number of new pain sites was lower in patients receiving therapy with 89-strontium [12].

Metastatic Spinal Cord Compression

Urgent treatment is required for metastatic spinal cord compression to avoid progression of motor deficits resulting in paraplegia. Early diagnosis and treatment are the 2 most important predictors of the final outcome of spinal cord compression. Radiotherapy and decompressive surgery are the most important treatment modalities. If the vertebral body has collapsed and bony fragments are impinging on the cord, surgical removal of the fragments and as much as possible of the tumor mass may benefit recovery.

Whether surgery or radiotherapy should be used as the initial treatment is still a matter of debate. The selection of the treatment is often influenced by prognostic factors like the presence of visceral metastases, the time period of developing motor deficits before treatment, the histology of the primary tumor, the interval from first diagnosis of cancer to metastatic spinal cord compression and the pretreatment ambulatory status.

A retrospective study from Denmark documented 398 cases with spinal cord compression due to metastatic lesions originating from different cancers, including prostate cancer in 19% of cases [13]. Patients treated by decompressive laminectomy followed by radiotherapy apparently had a better response than patients treated with surgery or irradiation alone, but when the patient's pretreatment motor function was taken into account, no significant difference was observed. Seventy-nine percent of the patients who were able to walk before treatment remained ambulatory, whereas only 18% of the nonambulatory patients regained walking ability.

A retrospective analysis of 1,304 patients with metastatic spinal cord compression and motor dysfunction of the lower extremities evaluated if there was a dependence of dose and fractionation in radiotherapy alone. In 1,304 patients (21% prostate cancer patients), it was found that the functional outcome was dose independent when comparing the different fractionation schedules (1 × 8, 5 × 4, 10 × 3, 15 × 2.5 and 20 × 2 Gy) [14]. Twenty-six percent of the patients who were not ambulatory before radiotherapy regained the ability to walk. Motor function improved in 26–31%. The more protracted schedules were associated with fewer in-field recurrences (7–14 vs. 24–26%, p < 0.001) and lower re-treatment rates. To minimize treatment time, the authors recommend a single fraction of 8 Gy for patients with poor predicted survival and 10 fractions of 3 Gy for all other patients.

Univariate analysis of the prognostic factors after radiotherapy of metastatic spinal cord compression showed improved local control was significantly associated with an absence of visceral metastases and long-course radiotherapy on multivariate analysis.

With regard to improved survival, histology, visceral metastases, other bone metastases, ambulatory status before radiotherapy, interval between tumor diagnosis and spinal cord compression as well as time of developing motor deficits, multivariate analysis showed significance [15].

Extracting the patients with metastatic spinal cord compression from patients arising from prostate cancer, Rades et al. [16] evaluated functional outcome and local control after radiotherapy, including a total of 281 patients. In that analysis, short-course (1 × 8 and 5 × 4 Gy) and long-course radiotherapy (10 × 3, 15 × 2.5 and 20 × 2 Gy) were compared [16]. The overall response to palliative radiotherapy was 86% (33% showed improvement of motor function, while 53% showed no further progression). Of the nonambulatory patients, 33% regained the ability to walk. On multivariate analysis, functional outcome was significantly affected by the time of developing motor deficits before radiotherapy (more than 14 days was better than 8–14 and 1–7 days, p < 0.001) and number of involved vertebrae (1–2 was better than ≥3, p = 0.013), but not by the radiation schedule (p = 0.859). The 2-year local control of metastatic spinal cord compression was 84%, depending on the radiation schedule (better after long-course radiotherapy, p = 0.001).

In conclusion, the functional outcome after palliative radiotherapy of metastatic spinal cord compression is significantly influenced by the time of developing motor deficits before radiotherapy and the number of involved vertebrae. Local control was significantly better after application of long-course radiotherapy. Patients with a poor expected survival could be treated with short-course radiotherapy to reduce the discomfort for the patient. For patients with good survival prognosis, long-course radiotherapy should be applied to achieve better local control.

Postoperative Palliative Radiotherapy

Postoperative radiotherapy following stabilizing surgical treatment is a standard procedure. It was shown that radiotherapy was the only significant predictor of normal use of the legs or arms after surgical intervention [17]. Except in patients with extremely bad prognosis, postoperative irradiation should be administered as a rule, especially with histologically proven residual tumor [18].

Symptomatic Local Progress

Local progressive prostate cancer can cause symptoms like perineal discomfort, urethral obstruction, pain and obstruction from invasion into the rectum, bleeding from the prostate or the urethra. Urinary retention can result in postrenal failure.

The application of a urethral catheter and analgesics are the first interventional procedures often necessary, followed by transfusions and transurethral resections of the prostate; cystostomy and nephrostomy are indicated in more locally advanced situations. Local irradiation for palliation is a noninvasive treatment promising reduction of the symptoms described above. It offers a relief of symptoms in most patients with hematuria, in up to 80% of patients with urinary outflow obstruction and in 50–70% of patients with pain secondary to locally advanced prostate carcinoma [19]. The local target volume should be restricted to the tumor itself, thus resulting in low rates of acute side effects occurring in the organs at risk.

Although palliative radiotherapy for local symptomatic progress is a widely used procedure, only few retrospective studies are available documenting the excellent palliative effect of radiotherapy. Complete symptomatic relief in 91% was documented by Ampil [20] in 20 patients given external beam irradiation because of malignancy-associated obstruction due to carcinoma of the cervix or prostate gland.

On local symptomatic progression of prostate cancer, Kawakami et al. [21] reported in 1993 that all patients with a urethral catheter were able to void without difficulty following treatment with local doses around 30 Gy and that all patients with severe hematuria responded completely. These effects lasted until patient death or for more than 11 months of follow-up [21].

These results were confirmed by Furuya et al. [22] in 1999, who presented data on the effects of radiotherapy on the local progression of hormone-refractory prostate cancer in 38 patients without distant progression. Of these, 11 patients were treated with local external beam radiotherapy at a dose of 50–66.6 Gy. Radiotherapy had a marked effect on symptoms associated with local progression

Moser/Schubert/Hinkelbein

and no patients suffered from symptoms after the radiotherapy. Complications of the treatment were frequent urination and diarrhea; however, no severe complications were observed. The local palliative effect was visible by shrinkage of the prostate by a mean of 14% following radiotherapy. Three- and five-year cause-specific survival rates were 46.2 and 22.1%, respectively [22].

The fractionation and dosage of external beam irradiation is debatable but always has to be adjusted to the patient's individual situation. In recent years, hypofractionated irradiation regimens were discussed for the curative treatment of prostate cancer. First results of single doses between 2.5 and 3 Gy up to total doses between 50 and 70 Gy showed promising results, with only high rates of acute side effects when single doses around 3 Gy were used [23–26]. For local palliation, hypofractionated schedules with total doses up to 50 or 60 Gy should be investigated, as they offer a reduced overall treatment time and may offer a long-lasting local palliative effect.

Conclusion

Radiotherapy has been a mainstay in the palliation of symptomatic metastatic prostate cancer and is most often used for palliation of painful metastatic bone lesions resulting in a relief of pain in about 80–90% of patients and therefore reduced dependence on analgesics.

In metastatic disease compromising the integrity of the spinal cord or a nerve root, radiotherapy can be used as an urgent intervention to minimize neurological dysfunction and local progression or as an adjunct to surgical decompression.

Local and systemic palliative treatment is always influenced by a patient's individual characteristics. As a component of the interdisciplinary cooperation, it is a challenge for the radiooncologist to optimize his treatment options according to the patient's individual situation. Radiotherapy is an effective local therapy, where some technical variables can and have to be adapted. The treatment volume, total dose and fractionation schedule depend, for example, on the patient's life expectancy, the likelihood of treatment success, the role of pharmacological intervention, the side effects of the treatment, the inconvenience of travelling to daily treatment sessions, the physical movement of men with unstable fractures onto and off the treatment tables, the disruption of hospice or other terminal care protocols and sometimes on the expense of treatment.

For progressive local and metastatic hormone-refractory prostate cancer, different systemic and local treatment options like analgesics, bisphosphonates, cytotoxic chemotherapy, hormone manipulation, radiotherapy and orthopedic interventions are available and often have to be combined, taking into account the individual palliative goals.

References

1 Bates T, Yarnold JR, Blitzer P, Nelson OS, Rubin P, Maher EJ: Bone metastases consensus statement. Int J Radiat Oncol Biol Phys 1992;23:215–216.

2 Gaze MN, Kelly CG, Kerr GR, Cull A, Cowie VJ, Gregor A, Howard GC, Rodger A: Pain relief and quality of life following radiotherapy for bone metastases: a randomized trial of two fractionation schedules. Radiother Oncol 1997;45:109–116.

3 Hartsell WF, Scott CB, Bruner DW, Scott CB, Bruner DW, Scarantino CW, Ivker RA, Roach M, Suh JH, Demas WF, Movsas B, Petersen IA, Konski AA, Cleeland CS, Janjan NA, DeSilvio M: Randomized trial of short- versus long-course radiotherapy for palliation of painful bone metastases. J Natl Cancer Inst 2005;97:798–804.

4 Jeremic B, Shibamoto Y, Acimovic L, Milicic B, Milisavljevic S, Nikolic N, Aleksandrovic J, Igrutinovic I: A randomized trial of three single-dose radiation therapy regimens in the treatment of metastatic bone pain. Int J Radiat Oncol Biol Phys 1998;42:161–167.

5 Koswig S, Budach V: Remineralization and pain relief in bone metastases after different radiotherapy fractions (10 × 3 vs. 1 × 8 Gy): a prospective study. Strahlenther Onkol 1999;175:500–508.

6 Nielsen OS, Bentzen SM, Sandberg E, Gadeberg CC, Timothy AR: Randomized trial of single dose versus fractionated palliative radiotherapy of bone metastases. Radiother Oncol 1998;47:233–240.

7 Niewald M, Tkocz HJ, Abel U, Scheib T, Walter K, Nieder C, Schnabel K, Berberich W, Kubale R, Fuchs M: Rapid course radiation therapy vs. more standard treatment: a randomized trial for bone metastases. Int J Radiat Oncol Biol Phys 1996;36:1085–1089.

8 Rasmusson B, Vejborg I, Jensen AB, Andersson M, Banning AM, Hoffmann T, Pfeiffer P, Nielsen HK, Sjogren P: Irradiation of bone metastases in breast cancer patients: a randomized study with 1 year follow-up. Radiat Oncol 1995;34:179–184.

9 Steenland E, Leer JW, van Houwelingen H, Post WJ, van den Hout WB, Kievit J, de Haes H, Martijn H, Oei B, Vonk E, van der Steen-Banasik E, Wiggenraad RG, Hoogenhout J, Warlam-Rodenhuis C, van Tienhoven G, Wanders R, Pomp J, van Reijn M, van Mierlo I, Rutten E: The effect of a single fraction compared to multiple fractions on painful bone metastases: a global analysis of the Dutch Bone Metastasis Study. Radiother Oncol 1999;52:101–109.

10 8 Gy single fraction radiotherapy for the treatment of metastatic skeletal pain: randomised comparison with a multifraction schedule over 12 months of patient follow-up. Bone Pain Trial Working Party. Radiother Oncol 1999;52:111–121.

11 Falkmer U, Järhult J, Wersäll P, Cavallin-Stahl E: A systematic overview of radiation therapy effects in skeletal metastases. Act Oncol 2003;42:620–633.

12 Quilty PM, Kirk D, Bolger JJ, Dearnaley DP, Lewington VJ, Mason MD, Reed NS, Russell JM, Yardley J: A comparison of the palliative effects of strontium-89 and external beam radiotherapy in metastatic prostate cancer. Radiother Oncol 1994;31:33–40.

13 Bach F, Larsen BH, Rohde K, Borgesen SE, Gjerris F, Boge-Rasmussen T, Agerlin N, Rasmusson B, Stjernholm P, Sorensen PS: Metastatic spinal cord compression: occurrence, symptoms, clinical presentations and prognosis in 398 patients with spinal cord compression. Acta Neurochir 1990;107:37–43.

14 Rades D, Stalpers LJA, Veninga T, Schulte R, Hoskin PJ, Obralic N, Bajrovic A, Rudat V, Schwarz R, Hulshof MC, Poortmans P, Schild SE: Evaluation of five radiation schedules and prognostic factors for metastatic spinal cord compression. J Clin Oncol 2005;23:3366–3375.

15 Rades D, Fehlauer F, Schulte R, Veninga T, Stalpers LJA, Basic H, Bajrovic A, Hoskin PJ, Tribius S, Wildfang I, Rudat V, Engenhart-Cabilic R, Karstens JH, Alberti W, Dunst J, Schild SE: Prognostic factors for local control and survival after radiotherapy of metastatic spinal cord compression. J Clin Oncol 2006;24:3388–3393.

16 Rades D, Stalpers LJ, Veninga T, Rudat V, Schulte R, Hoskin PJ: Evaluation of functional outcome and local control after radiotherapy for metastatic spinal cord compression in patients with prostate cancer. J Urol 2006;175:552–556.

17 Townsend PW, Rosenthal HG, Smalley SR, Cozad SC, Hassanein RE: Impact of postoperative radiation therapy and other perioperative factors on outcome after orthopedic stabilization of impending or pathologic fractures due to metastatic disease. J Clin Oncol 1994;12:2345–2350.

18 Schulte M, Hartwig E, Sarkar M, Arand M: Endoprostetic treatment of metastatic pathological fractures. Anticancer Res 1998;18:2251–2252.

19 Perez CA, Cosmatos D, Garcia DM, Eisbruch A, Poulter CA: Irradiation in relapsing carcinoma of the prostate. Cancer 1993;71(suppl):1110–1122.

20 Ampil FL: Radiation therapy palliation in malignancy-associated ureteral obstruction. Radiat Med 1989;7:282–286.

21 Kawakami S, Kawai T, Yamauchi T, Yonese J, Ueda T, Ishibashi K: Palliative radiotherapy for bone pain in hormone refractory prostate cancer. Nippon Hinyokika Gakkai Zasshi 1993;84:1681–1684.

22 Furuya Y, Akakura K, Akimoto S, Ichikawa T, Ito H: Radiotherapy for local progression in patients with hormone-refractory prostate cancer. Int J Urol 1999;6:187–191.

23 Livsey JE, Cowan RA, Wylie JP, Swindell R, Read G, Khoo VS, Logue JP: Hypofractionated conformal radiotherapy in carcinoma of the prostate: five-year outcome analysis. Int J Radiat Oncol Biol Phys 2003;57:1254–1257.

24 Akimoto T, Muramatsu H, Takahashi M, Saito J, Kitamoto Y, Harashima K, Miyazawa Y, Yamada M, Ito K, Kurokawa K, Yamanaka H, Nakano T, Mitsuhashi N, Niibe H: Rectal bleeding after hypofractionated radiotherapy for prostate cancer: correlation between clinical and dosimetric parameters and incidence of grade 2 or worse rectal bleeding. Int J Radiat Oncol Biol Phys 2004;60: 1033–1039.

25 Lukka H, Hayter C, Julian JA, Warde P, Morris WJ, Gospodarowicz M, Levine M, Sathya J, Choo R, Prichard H, Brundage M, Kwan W: Randomized trial comparing two fractionation schedules for patients with localized prostate cancer. J Clin Oncol 2005;23:6132–6138.

26 Kupelian PA, Thakkar VV, Khuntia D, Reddy CA, Klein EA, Mahadevan A: Hypofractionated intensity-modulated radiotherapy (70 Gy at 2.5 Gy per fraction) for localized prostate cancer: long-term outcomes. Int J Radiat Oncol Biol Phys 2005;63:1463–1468.

Dr. Lutz Moser
Klinik für Radioonkologie und Strahlentherapie, Charité Universitätsmedizin Berlin
Campus Benjamin Franklin, Hindenburgdamm 30
DE–12200 Berlin (Germany)
Tel. +49 30 8445 3051, Fax +49 30 8445 4463, E-Mail lutz.moser@charite.de

Author Index

Abrahamsson, P.-A. 1

Behmenburg, K. 93
Belka, C. 93
Boehmer, D. 26
Bottke, D. 32

Desgrandchamps, F. 86

Fosså, S.D. 108
Froehner, M. 39

Goldner, G. 68

Hakenberg, O.W. 39
Hinkelbein, W. 77, 117
Höcht, S. 77

Lohm, G. 77

Merseburger, A.S. 93
Miller, K. 7, 49
Moser, L. 77, 117

Pötter, R. 68

Rosewall, T. 15

Schostak, M. 7, 49
Schrader, M. 7, 49
Schubert, T. 117
Sia, M. 15
Stenzl, A. 93

Warde, P. 15
Wawroschek, F. 58
Wiegel, T. 32
Winter, A. 58
Wirth, M.P. 39
Wolff, J.M. 103

Subject Index

Active surveillance
  indications 3–5
  outcomes 3, 4
Aminoglutethimide, androgen-independent prostate cancer management 98
Androgen deprivation (AD)
  adjuvant hormonal treatment outcomes
    radical prostatectomy 40
    radiotherapy 40, 41
  age considerations 54
  Bicalutamide Early Prostate Cancer Program 43–46, 95, 96
  drugs, mechanisms, and side effects 27, 95, 96
  flutamide 96
  hormone-refractory disease, see Androgen-independent prostate cancer
  immediate initiation studies and survival outcomes 50, 51
  locally advanced prostate cancer, radical prostatectomy, and neoadjuvant therapy 11
  monotherapy for locally advanced or metastatic cancer 41–43
  neoadjuvant, concomitant, and adjuvant radiotherapy studies 27–29
  nilutamide 96
  prostate-specific antigen response 103, 104
  prostate volume effects 27, 29
  recurrence following radiotherapy management 87, 88
  risk stratification for external-beam radiotherapy and combination therapy
    intermediate-risk disease 18–20
    low-risk disease 17
  side effects and management 54, 55
  withdrawal response 95
Androgen-independent prostate cancer (AIPC)
  androgen depletion continuation in hormone-refractory prostate cancer 104
  androgen receptor-adapted therapy 99
  chemotherapy of hormone-refractory prostate cancer
    docetaxel 104
    docetaxel/estramustine 105, 106
    mitoxantrone/prednisone 105
    satraplatin 106, 107
  classification 94
  docetaxel/prednisolone study
    alkaline phosphatase response 115
    dosing 109, 110
    efficacy 110, 112–114
    patients 109–111
    prostate-specific antigen surge 114
    quality of life 110, 113
    safety and tolerability 113
    survival 113, 115
  palliative radiotherapy of symptomatic local progress 122, 123
  resistance development 93, 94

Androgen-independent prostate cancer
(AIPC) (continued)
secondary hormonal therapy
adrenal androgen inhibitors
aminoglutethimide 98
corticosteroids 97
ketoconazole 97
estrogens 98
progestins 98, 99
prospects 99
rationale in hormone-sensitive
prostate cancer 94, 95

Bicalutamide, *see* Androgen deprivation
Brachytherapy, *see* Radiotherapy

Chemotherapy
docetaxel/prednisolone for androgen-
independent prostate cancer
alkaline phosphatase response 115
dosing 109, 110
efficacy 110, 112–114
patients 109–111
prostate-specific antigen surge
114
quality of life 110, 113
safety and tolerability 113
survival 113, 115
hormone-refractory prostate cancer
docetaxel 104
docetaxel/estramustine 105, 106
mitoxantrone/prednisone 105
satraplatin 106, 107
recurrence following radiotherapy
management 90
Computed tomography (CT), lymph node
staging 59
Corticosteroids, androgen-independent
prostate cancer management 97
Cryotherapy, salvage therapy of recurrence
following radiotherapy 89
Cyproterone acetate, *see* Androgen
deprivation

Digital rectal examination (DRE)
recurrence evaluation 78
screening 2
Docetaxel, hormone-refractory prostate
cancer management 104

Docetaxel/estramustine, hormone-
refractory prostate cancer management
105, 106
Docetaxel/prednisolone, androgen-
independent prostate cancer study
alkaline phosphatase response 115
dosing 109, 110
efficacy 110, 112–114
patients 109–111
prostate-specific antigen surge 114
quality of life 110, 113
safety and tolerability 113
survival 113, 115

Estrogens, androgen-independent prostate
cancer management 98
External-beam radiotherapy, *see*
Radiotherapy

Flutamide, *see* Androgen deprivation

Goserelin, *see* Androgen deprivation

High-intensity focused ultrasound (HIFU),
salvage therapy of recurrence following
radiotherapy 90
Hormone-refractory disease, *see* Androgen-
independent prostate cancer
Hormone therapy, *see* Androgen
deprivation; Androgen-independent
prostate cancer

Ketoconazole, androgen-independent
prostate cancer management 97

Leuprorelin, *see* Androgen deprivation
Lycopene, recurrence following
radiotherapy management 90
Lymphadenectomy
pelvic lymph node dissection
techniques 60–62
therapeutic benefit 64
predictive nomograms 60
sentinel concept and relevance for
radiotherapy 64, 65
sentinel lymph node dissection 62–64
Lymph node staging
histopathological examination and effect
on detection rate 63

imaging 59
importance 52, 58, 59
predictive nomograms 60
prognostic value 52, 68, 69

Magnetic resonance imaging (MRI),
lymph node staging 59
Metastasis
consequences 52
hormone therapy 41–43
lymph node staging 52
palliative radiotherapy
skeletal metastases
external-beam irradiation
fractionation 118, 119
pain control 118
radionuclide therapy 119, 120
recalcification 119
toxicity 119
spinal cord compression 120, 121
Mitoxantrone/prednisone, hormone-
refractory prostate cancer management
105

Natural history, prostate cancer 2

Orchiectomy
disadvantages 50
prostate cancer growth effects 49, 95

Palliative radiotherapy, *see* Radiotherapy
Pelvic lymph node dissection, *see*
Lymphadenectomy
Polyestradiol phosphate, *see* Androgen
deprivation
Pomegranate juice, recurrence following
radiotherapy management 91
Positron emission tomography (PET),
lymph node staging 59
Progestins, androgen-independent prostate
cancer management 98, 99
Prostate-specific antigen (PSA)
androgen deprivation response 103,
104
docetaxel/prednisolone-induced surge
114
salvage radiotherapy guidance 79–82
screening 1, 2
tumor aggressiveness monitoring 53, 54

Prostate-specific membrane antigen,
radioimmunoscintigraphy 59

Radical prostatectomy
adjuvant hormonal treatment 40
age-dependent limits 50, 52
localized prostate cancer
complications 9
continence outcomes 4, 8
erectile function outcomes 4, 9
prognostic factors 8
locally advanced prostate cancer
continence outcomes 10
erectile function outcomes 10
neoadjuvant therapy
chemohormonal therapy 11
chemotherapy 11
hormone therapy 11
prognostic factors 9, 12
stage T3 cancer 10
margins 32, 33
postoperative adjuvant radiotherapy
acute and late side effects 36
pT2 tumors with positive margins
33, 34
pT3 tumors 34, 35
randomized trials 35, 36
radiotherapy in biochemical recurrence
after surgery 77–83
salvage therapy of recurrence following
radiotherapy 89
Radioimmunoscintigraphy, lymph node
staging 59
Radiotherapy
adjuvant hormonal treatment 40, 41
age considerations 52
complications 4
lymph node-positive cancer
disease control 71, 73, 76
patient characteristics 69–71
prognosis 68, 69, 73–75
side effects 70
study design 69, 70
survival 71–75
treatment planning 75
management of biochemical recurrence
after surgery 77–83
neoadjuvant, concomitant, and adjuvant
androgen deprivation studies 27–29

Radiotherapy (continued)
  palliative radiotherapy
    postoperative radiotherapy 122
    skeletal metastases
      external-beam irradiation
        fractionation 118, 119
      pain control 118
      radionuclide therapy 119, 120
      recalcification 119
      toxicity 119
    spinal cord compression 120, 121
    symptomatic local progress 122, 123
  postoperative adjuvant radiotherapy
    acute and late side effects 36
    pT2 tumors with positive margins
      33, 34
    pT3 tumors 34, 35
    randomized trials 35, 36
  recurrence following radiotherapy
    androgen depletion 87, 88
    chemotherapy 90
    definition 86
    evaluation 86, 87
    nonconventional therapies 90, 91
    salvage therapy
      brachytherapy 90
      cryotherapy 89
      high-intensity focused ultrasound
        90
      radical prostatectomy 89
    survival 87
  risk stratification for external-beam
    radiotherapy
    Genitourinary Radiation Oncologists
      of Canada system 16, 17
    high-risk disease 20, 22, 23
    intermediate-risk disease 18–20
    low-risk disease 17
  sentinel concept and relevance 64, 65

Satraplatin, hormone-refractory prostate
  cancer management 106, 107
Sentinel lymph node dissection, *see*
  Lymphadenectomy
SPCG-4, findings 2, 3
Spinal cord compression, palliative
  radiotherapy in metastasis 120, 121
Surgery, *see* Lymphadenectomy;
  Orchiectomy; Radical prostatectomy
Surveillance, *see* Active surveillance

Taxotere, *see* Docetaxel
Triptorelin, *see* Androgen deprivation

Ultrasonography, recurrence evaluation 78

Vitamin D, recurrence following
  radiotherapy management 91